Activities:
Reality and Symbol

Activities:
Reality and Symbol

Gail S. Fidler, OTR, FAOTA
Pompano Beach, Florida

Beth P. Velde, PhD, OTR/L
East Carolina University
Greenville, North Carolina

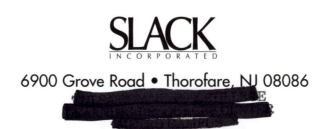

SLACK
INCORPORATED

6900 Grove Road • Thorofare, NJ 08086

Publisher: John H. Bond
Editorial Director: Amy E. Drummond
Associate Editor: Jennifer L. Stewart

Fidler, Gail S.
        Activities: Reality and symbol/Gail S. Fidler, Beth P. Velde.
          p. cm.
        Includes bibliographical references and index.
        ISBN 1-55642-383-7 (alk. paper)
    1. Occupational therapy--Symbolic aspects. 2. Occupational therapy--Social aspects. 3. Occupational therapy--Psychological aspects. I. Velde, Beth P. II. Title.
    RM735.F53   1999
    615.8'515--dc21

                                                                    98-45928
                                                                    CIP

For Library of Congress
Printed in the United States of America
Published by: SLACK Incorporated
                6900 Grove Road
                Thorofare, NJ 08086-9447 USA
                Telephone: 856-848-1000
                Fax: 856-853-5991
                http://www.slackinc.com

Last digit is print number: 10 9 8 7 6 5 4 3 2

DEDICATION

To the many colleagues and students who throughout my career have
stretched my learning. And most especially, to my husband Jay,
who during all these years has been my most valued teacher, mentor, and friend.
Gail S. Fidler

In appreciation for all they have taught me about the complexity
of human occupation and its role in quality of life, this book is dedicated to
my family and my students at College Misericordia and East Carolina University.
Beth P. Velde

A B O U T   T H E   C O V E R

The use of abstract art on the cover underscores the intent of this book: that objects, occupations, and behaviors manifest both real and symbolic messages. The reality of media choice, the uses and placement of colors, and patterns of brush strokes combine to present an actual art product. Simultaneously, the inherent abstraction of this presentation symbolically communicates and elicits both the artist's and the viewer's social, cultural, and personal ideations. Laughlin (1992), in his book titled *Brain, Symbol, and Experience: Towards a Neurophenomenology of Human Consciousness,* suggests that it is through contemplation of experience that the symbolic process occurs. We invite our readers to contemplate this piece of art and, thus, speculate on potential social and private meanings.

Laughlin, C. D. (1992). *Brain, symbol, and experience: Towards a neurophenomenology of human consciousness.* New York: Columbia University.

CONTENTS

CONTRIBUTING AUTHORS

Gail S. Fidler, OTR, FAOTA
Pompano Beach, Florida

Susan B. Fine, MA, OTR, FAOTA
Payne Whitney Psychiatric Clinic
New York Presbyterian Hospital
New York, New York

Beth P. Velde, PhD, OTR/L
East Carolina University
Greenville, North Carolina

P R E F A C E

This book describes the content and process for exploring and studying the social, cultural, and potential personal meanings inherent in activities. In our everyday lives, it is not uncommon for us to be made aware of an individual's affinity for or aversion to a particular activity. There are many examples demonstrating that a given activity can be enjoyable and gratifying to one person and boring or distasteful to another. Such dichotomy is evident in leisure and career pursuits, as well as in tasks of self-care and home maintenance.

A closer look at this phenomenon suggests that there is more to an explanation than talent and/or easy availability for involvement and learning. One is inevitably led to speculate about the possible dynamic of a congruence, or match, of an activity with the nature and characteristics of the person. If this is a credible hypothesis, then we can further postulate that to understand behavior, to comprehend the dynamics and impact of our nonhuman environment, we must come to know about the nature and dimensions of those activities that are such an inherent part of our environment and our lives.

Developing an understanding and indepth appreciation for the meanings of activities, their associated objects, and action processes is an essential prerequisite for using activities to promote health and enhance wellness and quality of life. It is imperative to the design of therapeutic and/or rehabilitative initiatives and/or to counsel toward pursuit of a productive, satisfying career.

This book, therefore, explores the characteristics of activities. It examines the potential of activities in their own right to represent, reflect, and infer social, cultural, and personal meanings and to communicate and call into play certain physical, affective, and cognitive responses. It is important to clarify that this is not a text about therapy or rehabilitation. The skills of application, of using activity or occupation in a curative process, can be mastered only to the extent of knowledge related to the complex dynamics of the characteristics of activities. The intent of this book is to initiate this learning and to guide the learner in exploring, discovering, and coming to know some of the dynamics of activities and their potential. This process certainly includes looking at and scrutinizing the relationship between an activity's characteristics and the behavioral responses most frequently elicited. However, attempting to extend these associations to therapeutic intervention is "jumping the gun." It risks distorting the focus of this study as well as doing an injustice to the complexities of therapeutic application.

The content of this book is organized to provide a sequential, experiential learning process of exploring, reflecting, speculating, and consensually validating experiences. To study activities means, of course, to experience activities. Thus, three very fundamental principles about learning are viewed as critical in studying the material presented in this work. These include the concept that new learning is integrated through the process of doing, through the active engagement of the learner. It should, therefore, be expected that discussions and analysis of the material presented here are preceded by relevant "doing" experiences. A second thesis relates to the importance of personal experience as the baseline for learning, for comparing and assessing, and for expanding perceptions and ideas. Thus, the learner's own experience should precede gathering information and impressions from others. Finally, the tempering of one's perceptions, clarification of one's thoughts, and the broadening of one's horizons evolves in large part from dialogue with others, from shared points of view, from explorations of differing opinions, and from arriving at a consensus about what is alike and what is different.

The development of the material in this book has evolved over time from such processes. It has been my privilege for many years to have had continued opportunities to dialogue with, share perspectives, and gain new insights from colleagues, students, friends, and clients. I am deeply indebted to these individuals who have made and continue to make my learning a richly rewarding experience.

This text can, in many ways, be characterized as a pursuit of meaning, an exploration of the many faces and voices, the doing experiences that comprise everyday life. Such a quest must rely heavily on the development and honing of creative problem-solving skills. This means to freely engage in associative and speculative thought, to guess outrageously, and to postpone the questions of validity and soundness until suppositions have been exhausted. We regularly make associations and assumptions regarding everyday encounters with events, people, and objects. We speculate on meaning, motives, and purpose. Now, students and teachers are asked to legitimize this process, to learn to apply it as access to new learning and new awareness.

Because this is an approach to learning uncharacteristic of traditional learning patterns, it is critically important to emphasize and practice this process as an integral approach to all material in this book. The questions raised in many of the chapters are there to stimulate uncensored associations and speculations. We need to remind ourselves that meaning is not absolute, neither are the dynamics of its unfolding. Questions such as "What comes to mind?" and "What might this mean?" are significant roadways on this journey to discovery.

The search to understand, the drive to learn, and the challenge of discovery are continual processes. This book represents some of what others and I know and are comfortable with hypothesizing about at this juncture. It is certainly not all that can be said, nor does it represent a final chapter. There is both challenge and satisfaction in knowing that tomorrows will bring new insights, new ideas, and new learning.

—Gail S. Fidler

Introductory Overview

Gail S. Fidler

The meaning and use of purposeful activity or occupation has been the hallmark of occupational therapy since its inception. Its history is replete with studies and discourses related to occupation, to purposeful activity as the core of the discipline. The major theories, frames of reference, and practice models of occupational therapy all address, from various perspectives, occupation or purposeful activity as fundamental in the study and practice of the profession. Cottrell (1996) offers an impressive collection of this profession's more recent literature addressing this topic. The disciplines of leisure studies and recreation, as well as psychology, have likewise explored the special roles that formalized activity plays in the health and welfare of individuals and society.

With such widespread consensus and study, it is striking to note the paucity of investigations and information regarding the inherent characteristics of activities, those elements that make up and define the nature of a given activity. There is significant information dealing with the physical, psychological, and social value of purposeful activity and occupation; however, the breadth and depth of study regarding the symbolic and realistic characteristics of activities in and of themselves within a cultural, social, and personal context is markedly limited. Much of the literature related to this realm of study deals mostly with the instrumental and sociological characteristics of an activity in contrast to the inherent metaphors and symbolic aspects. There are some exceptions, of course, the more recent and notable ones being

Bettleheim (1977), Brunner (1990), Csikszentmihalyi (1990), Csikszentmihalyi and Rochberg-Halton (1981; and several of the papers published in the Zemke and Clark (1996) volume. Also, see Chapter 3.

The discipline of therapeutic recreation emphasizes the inclusion of meaningful leisure activities as part of the total life experience (Peterson & Gunn, 1984). The associated field of leisure education attempts to provide individuals with the knowledge to choose leisure activities that are personally meaningful and purposeful (Howe-Murphy & Charboneau, 1987).

There appears to be an increasing interest in the field of nursing regarding purposeful activity. Holistic nursing textbooks include chapters that discuss the interrelationship of the environment and activity, activities that result in play and laughter, relaxation, and music. The self-assessments included in such texts address behaviors related to health and the balance between work-related, personal, and play activities (Dossey, Keegan, Guzzetta, & Kolkmeier, 1995).

When our principle concern is the art and science of "doing," of enabling a sustained engagement in those activities, those occupations that comprise a personally relevant lifestyle that is satisfying to self and others, the dynamics of what enables such engagement becomes a fundamental question. The first step in understanding this phenomenon is to come to know the salient characteristics of activities, their properties, and the social, cultural, and personal realities and symbolic inferences of these.

To pursue this journey requires coming to appreciate that an activity, an occupation, has meaning in its own right (Csikszentmihalyi & Rochberg-Halton, 1981; Fidler & Fidler, 1963). This involves understanding that it is the unique nature and characteristic of an activity that influences and shapes the motivational and behavioral responses of the performer. Furthermore, the characteristic of an activity or occupation and the performance of an individual in that activity, although related, are two quite distinct aspects (Fidler & Fidler, 1963; Nelson, 1988). The match, or congruence, between person and activity is the dynamic that triggers motivation and sustains engagement (Csikszentmihalyi, 1990; Fidler & Fidler, 1978). Developing a sophisticated understanding of the unique qualities of activities is one side of the coin. The other side is, of course, knowing the person, understanding human psychology.

Before moving forward in this exploration, it is important to clarify what we mean when we use the term "an activity."

An activity and an occupation are used interchangeably in this text. Each is understood and defined as a sphere or set of interdependent actions that require the active engagement of an individual's mind and body in pursuit of the intended outcome or end product of that sphere or set of actions. Similarly, Webster (1991) defines an activity as comprising the pursuit of an outcome involving mental function and vigorous or energetic action. A task is viewed as part of an activity, a segment of an action set. I suggest that the elements of an activity or occupation include the following:

- *Structure and form:* The required rules, procedures, time element, and standards.
- *Physical properties:* The essential objects, materials, and setting.
- *Action processes:* The psychomotor behaviors required in relation to the use of form and properties.
- *Outcome:* The discernable results or end product of the activity.
- *The realistic and symbolic dimensions of the activity's social, cultural, and personal meanings:* Of the total activity or occupation as well as each of its parts (structure, properties, action, and outcome).

Each of these are explored throughout this book, and Chapter 5 presents an organized process for analyzing each of these categories.

Csikszentmihalyi and Rochberg-Halton (1981) assert that,

Humans display the intriguing characteristic of making and using objects. The things with which people interact are not simply tools for survival, or for making survival easier and more comfortable. Things embody goals, they make skills manifest and shape the identity of their users. Man is not only homo sapiens or homo ludens, he is also homo faber, the maker and user of objects. This self to a large extent is a reflection of things with which he interacts. Thus objects also make and use their makers and users! (p. 11)

The social, cultural, and personal meanings and metaphors inherent in an activity are an essential aspect of understanding purposeful activity. Because of our ability as humans to abstract, we are able to think symbolically. Thus, events, activities, and objects, in addition to being signs or having a specific reality, take on certain connotations representing concepts that relate to all aspects of human activity. The advertising industries understand this quite well. The popular ads for jeans, perfumes, aftershave lotions, and sneakers are only a few examples of the ubiquitous use of symbols and symbolic thought in daily life. Realistic is a relatively easy concept to grasp. What is real, what is actual, can be seen, agreed upon, and precisely named. A baseball, basketball, hair brush, or pine tree, for example, bring to mind for each of us the same object. They exist in fact. However, if we ask what each of these mean, the question becomes complex. We begin to enter the realm of symbolism and symbolic subjective thought. It is important to understand the distinction between symbol and sign. A sign indicates the existence of a thing, an event, or condition. It is a concrete "in place of" an event, object, or condition. Thus, a wet road is a sign that it has rained, a red traffic light means stop, green means go. A sign is directly translatable, a concrete representation (Plokker, 1964).

A symbol is far more complex; it is not a proxy for its object, condition, or event. It is a "carrier" of a concept; it conveys a meaning; it communicates a thought, an abstract idea. Symbols always contain an affective element. These vary according to cultures and individuals. There are symbols that are universal, culturally specific, and/or idiosyncratic (Csikszentmihalyi, 1990; Jung, 1964). Universal symbols are those that have the same or a similarly generalized meaning across cultures. Objects such as the sun, moon, wind, rain, food, and God are such examples. Culturally specific symbols are those that communicate, that convey meanings specific to a given culture. The horseshoe, wishbone, football, rosary, icons, hex signs, and four-leaf clover are such examples. Idiosyncratic or personal symbols are those that convey one's personal feelings, concepts, and associations. They carry particular personal meanings. For example, a basketball may be perceived realistically as a particular kind of ball used in a definable, organized, competitive game. It may also be personally symbolic of success or failure to one person, convey messages about social structure and strategy to another, or be symbolic of ineptness, competence, parental expectations, or peer judgments to others. Following a pattern, cutting on a line, sanding a board, or operating a word processor may have meaning, as these endeavors realistically relate to accomplishing a given task or activity, producing an end product, mastering or learning a particular skill. Such activity may also symbolize and, thus, embody personal attitudes, feelings, and abilities with regard to, for example, doing what is expected, complying and "towing the line," or controlling, being aggressive or ordering one's world, manipulating or shaping one's environment, and being an agent or a cause.

How one's culture views, for example, carpentry, construction, and basketball, the gender roles, and required psychomotor behavior in relation to these has, of course, a significant impact on personal meanings. Understanding the meaning of the experience for any given individual, thus, requires knowing both levels of the activity: the realistic and the symbolic. Csikszentmihalyi and Rochberg-Halton (1981) remind us that, "one of the most important but unfortunately most neglected aspects of the meaning of things is precisely the ability of an object to convey meaning through its own inherent qualities" (p. 43).

We can learn a great deal from anthropology about the reality base and symbolic meanings of activities, objects, and action processes, and how these both reflect and shape human existence and society. There is a wealth of information about ritual objects and activities in both primitive and sophisticated societies, which is essential to the understanding of human performance (Campbell, 1962; Langer, 1956). Fairy tales are also an excellent example of the social and personal uses of both real and symbolic "messages." What are the messages, the connotations, for example, of the tales and rhymes of Little Boy Blue, Walt Disney's Pocahontas, Ninja Turtles, the Power Rangers, or Superman? All of art, drama, sports, games, jobs, and careers provide multidimensional experiences and learning at both a realistic and symbolic level. These trigger the critical interplay of mind and body so essential to the integration of our internal systems, while simultaneously being agents of our socialization, our relatedness to the external world.

Read (1970) has explained how art teaches fundamental functions through eliciting the engagement of sensory, motor, and cognitive functions. He views education related to visual arts, design, and architecture as training the eye to see and perceive beyond the obvious. The plastic arts, such as ceramics and sculpture, are seen as educating and developing the sense and skills of touch. Musical education, such as learning to play an instrument and/or listening to music, is considered significant in developing a sophisticated ear, an ability to hear beyond sound. Learning in the verbal arts, such as drama and poetry, Read contends, teaches the skills of speech and articulation, and education related to crafts and construction activities stimulates and develops cognitive functions, the orderly processes of thought.

Those of us who have used object histories as a learning experience for students have come to appreciate more fully the significance of a person's attachment to nonhuman objects. A description of the object history is included in Chapter 4. Use of the object history over time has shown how engagement with objects (one's object relationship) provides learning and exploration. It portrays the ways in which these experiences enable organization and integration of sensorimotor, psychological, and cognitive processes and how such engagement nurtures and shapes feelings, attitudes, values, and interpersonal potential. Through such exploration, it has been possible to obtain a glimpse of the ways in which the dynamics of object relationships are related to characteristic play experiences, to the formation of adult activity patterns, to ways of coping, and to strategies of adaptations. Object histories, furthermore, provide a unique opportunity to compare and study social and cultural differences, for example in the choice of objects, how they are used, as well as the varying social roles, values, and behaviors that are taught and reinforced through the activity. These themes are explored in a number of studies including Csikszentmihalyi and Rochberg-Halton (1981), Erikson (1971), and Searles (1962). My collection of students' object histories over several decades has been a rich resource for such learning.

Play histories (Fidler, 1971; Takata, 1971) add to this exploration, reflecting cultural differences in the choice of games and play as well as in the variations of rules and procedures. For example, rope jumping, popular among girls during puberty and very early adolescence, obviously reflects and is responsive to the kind and level of their physical maturation. The rhymes that are such an inherent part of this activity are metaphors of the expectations (personal and social) of what becoming a woman is all about. Gender role learning is extended and reinforced through traditional activities and object relationships with the Barbie doll, baby dolls, playing house, nurse or doctor, eye-hand coordinating activities, TV commercials, and cheerleader dress and activity.

Baseball and similar sports and group games characteristic of the activity of boys at the age of puberty and early adolescence are congruent with their level of physical maturation and, thus, provide opportunities for skill development. Realistically and symbolically, these activities provide social role learning about teamwork, competition, aggression, and confrontation. Role values and behaviors are further developed in the growing boy through his engagement with traditional toys, such as guns, swords, fire engines, cars, the Power Rangers, Ninja Turtles, television commercials, films, sports heroes, and the computer. The more recent introduction of team sports and the world of computer activities among young girls can be expected over time to change the socialization of women. Observing and studying such change should provide us with additional evidence of how activities both reflect and shape human values, attitudes, and behaviors.

We need only to observe the kind of activities that characterize our world of today to sense the social meaning and significance of activities. Organized national sports and related industries, marathons, television sagas of aggression and violence, television and print advertising, and the Internet enable us to make some speculations about how activities both reflect national values, themes, and agendas and are, in turn, influenced by them. Throughout civilization, activities have been used to teach at both a realistic and symbolic level—those attitudes, morals, skills, and behaviors relative to what is necessary for survival and adaptation. Greek literature, mythology, anthropology, histories of civilization, the arts, philosophy, and religion all address these themes in various ways. One very relevant illustration of the use of the symbolic aspects of activities to teach coping skills has come from the work of Moore and Anderson (1968). Their research proposed that in all cultures, primitive or sophisticated, the process of humanization is generated by engagement in four categories of activities. These encompass puzzles that teach agency skills and roles, games of chance that teach the recipient role, games of strategy that enable learning about the importance of the significant other, and aesthetic processes that teach the role of judge or referee. Not only have these scientists related specific elements of games and activities to the necessary perspectives and skills required for dealing with the most significant features of a society's relationship with its environment, but their principles for designing a responsive, clarifying environment comprises a useful, activity-based paradigm. More recently, Cynkin and Robinson (1990) and others have described how activities are socioculturally regulated by a system of values, beliefs, and customs and are, thus, defined by them, which, in turn, define acceptable norms of behavior.

I have hypothesized (Fidler, 1981) that the relative meaning and significance of an activity or occupation is measured by the value judgments of society, the person-activity congruence, the activity's integrative potential, and the verifiability of its end product. The match of person to an activity, the congruence between the salient characteristics of an activity, and the biopsychosocial characteristics of the person are critical variables in understanding individual intrinsic motivation, gratification, and the experience of success.

The rope jumping skills of the young girl, the positive responses to the proprioceptive input and social relevance of volleyball for the adolescent and young adult, and the gross motor coordination skills and high energy level of an individual who makes soccer an intrinsically gratifying success experience illustrates this thesis. It is acknowledged, for example, that defensive football players have a neuro-psychology, a sensorimotor organization, and a response pattern different from those who become successful offensive team members. The perceptual neuro-motor requirements for being a wide receiver are quite different from those required of the middle linebacker. The performance imperatives of print journalism are different from those of sculpting or bookkeeping. How might, for example, the differences and similarities among the following be described?

- Stamp collecting, murder mystery reading, and chess?
- Football, baseball, tennis, skiing?
- Monopoly, crossword puzzles, black jack, Trivial Pursuit?
- Sculpting, knitting, typing, cooking?
- Middle linebacker, wide receiver, goalie, pitcher?

The extent to which we find our jobs or hobbies enjoyable is the extent to which there is a match between our sensorimotor, cognitive, psychological, and interpersonal characteristic, our social and cultural orientation, and the characteristics (realistically and symbolically) of the job or hobby. It is this congruence, this match of person characteristics and activity characteristics that triggers and sustains intrinsic motivation. Inherent in such a match is continuity, the ongoing incentive to maintain such engagement. We speak of a chemistry between people and call it love. There is ample evidence of chemistry between person and activity, and Csikszentmihalyi (1990) calls it *flow*!

The following chapters in this book explore some of the dynamics that make that chemistry possible.

The significance of engagement in activities and the value that such involvement has in sustaining health and a sense of well-being, in shaping the quality of one's living and as a therapeutic and rehabilitative endeavor, is universally recognized. The extensive studies and promotion of leisure and recreation, the universal popularity of sports and games, the study and application of the creative arts and recreation in treatment, and the growth of occupational therapy all offer ample evidence of a powerful belief in the efficacy of activities.

REFERENCES

Bettleheim, B. (1977). *The use of enchantment: The meaning and importance of fairy tales*. New York: Knopf.

Campbell, J. (1962). *The masks of god: Primitive mythology* (vol. 1). New York: Viking.

Cottrell, R. (Ed.) (1996). *Purposeful activity: Foundation & future of occupational therapy*. Bethesda, MD: American Occupational Therapy Association.

Csikszentmihalyi, M. (1990). *Flow: The psychology of optimal experience*. New York: Harper Row.

Csikszentmihalyi, M., & Rochberg-Halton, E. (1981). *The meaning of things: Domestic symbols and the self*. Cambridge, MA: Cambridge University Press.

Cynkin, S. & Robinson, A. (1990). *Occupational therapy and activities health*. Boston: Little, Brown & Co.

Dossey, B. M., Keegan, L., Guzzetta, C. E., & Kolkmeier, L. G. (1995). *Holistic nursing: A handbook for practice* (2nd ed.). Gaithersburg, MD: Aspen Publishers.

Erikson, E. (1971). *Toys and reason: Stages in the ritualization of experience*. New York: W. W. Norton.

Erikson, E. H. (1976). Play and actuality. In: J. S. Brunner. *Play, its role in development and evolution*. New York: Basic Books.

Fidler, G. S. (1971). *The play history*. Unpublished outline.

Fidler, G. S. (1981). From crafts to competence. *Am J Occup Ther, 35,* 567-573.

Fidler, G. S. (1988). *Supplementary information for examining the knowledge base of occupational therapy*. American Occupational Therapy Foundation. Unpublished paper.

Fidler, G. S., & Fidler, J. W. (1963). *Occupational therapy: A communication process in psychiatry*. New York: MacMillan.

Fidler, G. S., & Fidler, J. W. (1978). Doing and becoming: Purposeful action and self actualization. *Am J Occup Ther, 32,* 305-310.

Howe-Murphy, R., & Charboneau, B. G. (1987). *Therapeutic recreation intervention: An ecological perspective*. Englewood Cliffs, NJ: Prentice-Hall.

Jung, C. (1964). *Man and his symbols*. New York: Doubleday.

Langer, S. K. (1956). *Philosophy in a new key: Study in symbolism of reason, rite and art*. New York: Mentor.

Moore, O. K., & Anderson, A. R. (1968). *Some principles for the design of clarifying educational environments*. Pittsburgh: University of Pittsburgh Press.

Nelson, G. (1988). Occupation: Form and performance. *Am J Occup Ther, 42,* 632-641.

Peterson, C. A., & Gunn, S. L. (1984). *Therapeutic recreation program and design: Principles and procedures* (2nd Ed.). Englewood Cliffs, NJ: Prentice-Hall.

Plokker, J. H. (1964). *Art from the mentally disabled*. Boston: Little, Brown & Co.

Read, H. (1970). *Education through art*. London: The Shenvel Press.

Searles, H. (1962). *The non-human environment*. New York: International Universities Press.

Takata, N. (1971). The play milieu: A preliminary appraisal. *Am J Occup Ther, 25,* 281-285.

Webster (1991). *Ninth New Collegiate Dictionary*. Springfield, MA: Merriam Webster.

Zemke, R. & Clark, F. (1996). Occupational science: The evolving discipline. Philadelphia: F. A. Davis.

ADDITIONAL READING

Arieti, S. (1967). *The intrapsychic self*. New York: Basic Books.

Arieti, S. (1976). *Creativity: The major synthesis*. New York: Basic Books.

Avedon, E., & Sutton-Smith, B. (1971). *The study of games*. New York: John Wiley and Sons.

Benedict, R. (1934). *Patterns of culture*. Boston: Houghton Mifflin.

Brunner, J. S. (1962). *On knowing: Essays for the left hand*. Cambridge, MA: Belknap Press.

Brunner, J. (1972). The nature and uses of immaturity. *Am Psych, 27,* 687-708.

Brunner, J. (1990). *Acts of meaning*. Cambridge, MA: Harvard University Press.

Brunner, J., Jolly, A., & Silva, K. (Eds.) (1976). *Play: its role in development and evolution*. New York: Basic Books.

Bulfinch, T. *Bulfinches mythology: The age of fable: The age of chivalry: The legends of Charlemagne*. New York: Modern Library.

Coelho, G., Hamburg, D. T., & Adams, J. (Eds.). (1974). *Coping and adaptation*. New York: Basic Books.

Csikszentmihalyi, M. (1975). *Beyond boredom and anxiety*. San Francisco: Jossey-Bass.

Csikszentmihalyi, M. (1976). What play says about behavior. *Ontario Psychologist, 8,* 5-11.

Deci, E. L., & Ryan, P. M. (1985). *Intrinsic motivation and self determination in human behavior*. New York: Plenum Press.

Fidler, G. S. (1968). The task oriented group as a context for treatment. *Am J Occup Ther, 23,* 43-48.

Fidler, G. S. (1982). The activity laboratory: A structure for observing and assessing perceptual, integrative and behavioral strategies. In: B. Hemphill (Ed.). *The evaluative process in psychiatric occupational therapy*. Thorofare, NJ: SLACK, Incorporated.

Fidler, G. S., & Fidler, J. W. (1983). Doing and becoming. The occupational therapy experience. In G. Kielhofner (Ed.), *Health through occupation: Theory and practice in occupational therapy*. Philadelphia: F. A. Davis.

Fidler, G. S., & Ridgway, E. (1955). *Occupational therapy: Laboratory for living*. Mental Health Views #3. Philadelphia: Office of Health Education. Department of Public Health.

Fine, S., & Fidler, G. S. (1971). *The object history*. Unpublished outline.

Fontana, D. (1994). *The secret language of symbols*. San Francisco: Chronicle Books.

Geertz, E. (1971). *The interpretation of cultures*. New York: Basic Books.

Godbey, G. (1991). *Leisure in your life: An application* (3rd ed.). State College, PA: Ventura Publishing, Inc.

Goldschmidt, W. (1974). Ethology, ecology and ethnological realities. In G. V. Coelho, D. A. Hamburg, & J. E. Adams (Eds.). *Coping and adaptation*. New York: Basic Books.

Greenberg, P. F. (1977). The thrill seekers. *Human Behavior, 6,* 17-21.

Hall, E. T. (1959). *The silent language*. New York: Doubleday.

Hall, J. (1974). *Dictionary of subjects and symbols in art*. London: John Murray Press.

Ibrahim, H. (1991). *Leisure and society: A comparative approach*. Madison, WI: W. C. Brown.

Kelly, J. (1987). *Freedom to be: A new sociology of leisure*. New York: MacMillan.

Kelly, J., & Goodboy, G. (1992). *The sociology of leisure*. State College, PA: Ventura Publishing.

Kielhofner, G. (1985). *A model of human occupation: Theory and application*. Baltimore: Williams and Wilkins.

Kielhofner, G. (1997). *Conceptual foundation of occupational therapy*. Philadelphia: F. A. Davis.

King, L. J. (1978). Toward a science of adaptive responses. *Am J Occup Ther, 32,* 429-437.

Lever, J. (1978). Sex differences in the complexity of children's play. *American Sociological Review, 84,* 471-483.

Mead, M. (1928). *Coming of age in Samoa*. New York: Morrow.

Mecanic, D. (1974). Social structure and personal adaptation: Some neglected dimensions. In G. V. Coelho, D. A. Hamburg, & J. E. Adams (Eds.). *Coping and Adaptation*. New York: Basic Books.

Pribram, K. H. (1971). *Language of the brain*. Englewood Cliffs, NJ: Prentice Hall.

Provost, J. (1990). *Work, play and type: Achieving balance in your life*. Palo Alto, CA: Psychologists' Press.

Reilly, M. (Ed.) (1974). *Play as exploratory learning*. Beverly Hills, CA: Sage Publications.

Robinson, A. L. (1977). The arena for acquisition of rules for competent behavior. *Am J Occup Ther, 11,* 248-253.

Rochberg-Halton, E. (1979). The meaning of personal art objects. In J. Zazawak (Ed.). *Social research and cultural policy*. Waterloo: Otium Publications.

Shannon, P. (1977). The derailment of occupational therapy. *Am J Occup Ther, 31,* 229-234.

Shapiro, D. (1982). *Loss, motivation and activity in bereavement of the physically disabled*. New York: Arno Press.

Sherman, E., & Newman, E. S. (1977). The meaning of cherished personal possessions for the elderly. *Journal of Aging and Human Development, 8,* 181-192.

Shweder, R. A., & LeVine, R. A. (Eds.) (1984). Culture theory: Essays on mind, self and emotion. New York: Cambridge University Press.

Turner, V. W. (1967). *The forest of symbols*. Ithaca, NY: Cornell University Press.

Vroom, J. (1995). *Work and motivation*. San Francisco: Jossey-Bass.

White, R. (1974). Strategies of adaptation: An attempt at systematic description. In G. V. Coelho, D. A. Hamburg, & J. E. Adams. *Coping and adaptation*. New York: Basic Books.

Williamson, G. (1872). A heritage of activity: Development of theory. *Am J Occup Ther, 36,* 716-722.

Yerxa, E. (1967). Authentic occupational therapy. *Am J Occup Ther, 21,* 1-9.

CHAPTER 2

Symbolization: Making Meaning for Self and Society

Susan B. Fine

INTRODUCTION

If we hope to live not just from moment to moment, but in true consciousness of our existence, then our greatest need and most difficult achievement is to find meaning in our lives. (Bettelheim, 1977, p. 3)

In a society that increasingly defines itself on the basis of behaviorism ("What you see is what you get") and materialism ("What you have is who you are"), the search for "meaning," in its more substantive sense, is most often relegated to philosophers, social scientists, or religious scholars. However, meaning and the phenomena that influence it deeply affect the integrity of each individual and society at large. Bettelheim's existential reflections, in fact, address an imposing human capacity that we employ with regularity. Although we may not always be aware of this tendency, we appraise and seek meaning in a multitude of situations and activities: those we initiate and those to which we respond. We choose to play a mournful recording again and again because the words, the vocalist, and the rhythms touch us deeply. We ruminate about whether the changes in our worksite are a threat or an opportunity. We look at old photographs because they recapture our past and help define us. We puzzle over the residual feelings of a recurring dream. We look for causes in the attitudes of friends or family members. We have a compelling need "to know," and we pursue those needs through sensation, thoughts, emotion, or, more accurately, the integrative activities of mind, brain, and environment.

The often cryptic nature of the meaning-seeking process is one of its most valuable qualities, because authentic meaning only declares itself in the life context of a given individual or a particular social group. The favored love song of one person may seem irrelevant to another. The loss of a pet may be deeply tragic to some, but only a sad milestone for others. While there are predictable themes that define and challenge human existence, there is no prescription for determining meaningfulness. We seek it through our unique biopsychosocial filter—and if we fail to find an adequate source in reality, we frequently invent it!

The activities that characterize the reality of our daily lives—the obligatory, the chosen, the serendipitous—are a reflection of our personal and cultural "inventiveness." How each of us imbues and explains them is often of greater importance than their reality. *Personal perspective* influences what we value and choose to do, the quality of our engagement, the satisfaction we experience, and the effectiveness of the outcome. Seeking and finding meaning in ourselves, our activities, and the broader world of people and things around us is a remarkable, but often undervalued, gift that permits adaptation and growth for both the individual and society.

There are many biological, psychological, and sociocultural elements that promote this phenomena. These domains will be explored throughout this book, an endeavor that pays tribute to the richness and significance of activities. One cannot, however, pursue this ambitious project without first acknowledging some charismatic and indispensable tools for "meaning making": *symbols* and the *symbolization process*. That is the task of this chapter.

Basic Assumptions: Meaning and the Inner Life

The material in this chapter is informed by two basic and essential assumptions. The first, the aforementioned belief that *there is a unique human need to understand and give meaning to our experiences*, is a legacy of many social and neuroscientists, art historians, theologians, and philosophers (Bruner, 1990; Cirlot, 1962; Csikszentmihalyi & Rochberg-Halton, 1981; Edelman, 1992; Freud, 1955; Jung, 1964; Kleinman, 1988; Lazarus & Folkman, 1984; Sacks, 1964; Turner, 1988; Vaillant, 1993). While their belief systems and applications are diverse and sometimes conflicting, they share a conviction about the important role that meaning assumes in the everyday routine, in the circumstances of traumatic life events, and in the unfolding life stages of the individual and his or her culture. In this tradition, the evolving interdisciplinary science of occupation (Zemke & Clark, 1996) has focused attention on the ways in which meaningful "chunks of daily activity that can be named in the lexicon of the culture" (p. IX) influence health and the construction of individual identities. The reader is encouraged to investigate these and other references cited at the end of this chapter. They provide a valuable foundation for understanding the symbolization process and Fidler's beliefs about *the dynamic chemistry between people and activities.*

The second key postulate involves *the acknowledgement of the "inner life"*—those mental processes that deal with thoughts and feelings and influence consciousness and behavior. This includes those unconscious processes originally associated with Freudian theories of conflict and repression.

The "unconscious" ... is indeed a marvelous metaphoric organ. With its ebb and flow of emotion, its stored record of salient experience, its concourse with the body and its well-blazed trails of feeling and expression, it can generate dreams, errors, beliefs, symptoms, lifelong patterns of word and deed, while its mechanisms remain unbeknownst to us. (Konner, 1982, p. 180)

Ego psychology has expanded the antecedents to behavior beyond Freud's instinctual drives, refining and redirecting the promise of the unconscious and conflict-free ego functions (Vaillant, 1993), while neuroscience has demystified their metaphoric status by identifying patterns of brain activity that work outside the realm of conscious awareness to contain events, thoughts, and feelings that threaten the self-concept (Edelman, 1992; Gazzaniga, 1988). Gazzaniga's concept of the left-brain's interpretive role in mental activities serves to enhance our understanding of the interactive relationships between mind and brain and the complex ways in which "brain mechanics are tied to our seemingly highly personal mind mechanics" (p. 4). These brain patterns, derived from the emotion-laden memories they support, from our current relationships with the external environment, as well as from evolutionary effects of man's involvement in preferred activities (Zemke & Clark, 1996), influence the form and substance of the messages emerging in dreams, the creative work of artists, religious rituals, and the language of everyday life.

Not all advocates of contemporary science, however, support the affective richness of the inner life. There is an unfortunate tendency, in the so-called cognitive revolution, to reduce the mind to an information processing system "... disconnected from experience, historical and cultural factors, and the ... background context in which particular actions or thought occur" (Vaillant, 1993, p. 4). For some readers, as well, pursuit of the inner life may require an extraordinary act of faith, because society continues to devalue the introspective, or what may be perceived to be "psychoanalytic." Acknowledging the unconscious inner life in the context of today's dynamic biopsychosocial dialectic does not commit one to the couch. It simply, and profoundly, opens the door to *a fuller understanding of how human activities at one level influence processes at another.* Exploring it is well worth the risk!

Symbolism: Mind over Matter

Man, it has been said, is a symbolizing animal. Science and technology have not freed [him] from his dependence on symbols; indeed, it may be argued that they may have increased his need for them. (Read, 1962, p. IX)

Read's characterization captures the critical interplay and tension between prevailing human needs, civilization's development and discontents, and the role symbols play in mediating between the two. It is, in fact, *the duality* of the symbol—the implication of there being more than what appears to be; the latent as well as the manifest—that empowers it to fulfill its core purpose: *connecting the inner life and the consciousness of the individual with the collective belief systems of his or her culture.*

A symbol has been defined as "a term, a name, or even a picture that may be familiar in daily life, yet that possesses specific connotations in addition to its conventional and obvious meaning" (Jung, 1964, p. 20). This capacity to connote *something more* distinguishes symbols from the less complex representational function of signs. The latter simply designate objects to which they may be arbitrarily attached (i.e., the National Organization for Women [NOW] and traffic signs), while the dynamism of the symbol rests in its ability to simultaneously express the various aspects of the idea it represents, or the total experience of the person engaged in the symbolization process.

The word *symbol* comes from the Greek *sym* plus *bollein*: to "throw together," to unite (Csikszentmihalyi & Rochberg-Halton, 1981). It is "... a bringing together, into a meaningful pattern, of the person's experience on many different levels—unconscious and conscious, historical and present, sensual and intellectual, social and individual" (May, 1968, p. 15). This process is aptly described by the late Nobel Prize-winning poet Octavio Paz:

> *Between what I see and what I say*
> *Between what I say and what I keep silent*
> *Between what I keep silent and what I dream*
> *Between what I dream and what I forget:*
> Poetry (New York Times, April 25, 1998, p. 1)

Symbols are everywhere—in the colloquialisms of the street as well as in the poet's lyrical choice of words, in the art and music we create, in the gestures we make, in the clothing in which we present ourselves, in the dreams we have, and in the objects with which we surround ourselves. They may be consciously and carefully chosen, as in the writing of advertising copy; they may be unconscious and spontaneous, emerging in a dream or linked to an object in our environment; or they may spring from an amalgam of both, as sometimes occurs when the sculptor transforms a lump of clay or a congregant participates in a religious service. Its ubiquitous nature is evident in the history of mankind as well as in the life of each person and his or her contemporaneous social group.

Historical Perspectives

Symbolism has a long and enduring history that is woven throughout the development of man in both Eastern and Western cultures (Cirlot, 1962; Jung, 1964). Most writers agree that the beginnings of symbolist thought can be found in prehistoric times—in the latter part of the Paleolithic Age when the stars, animals, plants, stones, and other aspects of nature were ancient man's teachers.

> *The process whereby the beings of this world are ordered according to their properties, so that the words of action and of spiritual and moral facts may be explored by analogy ... can be seen ... in the transition from the pictograph into the ideograph as well as in the origins of art.* (Cirlot, 1962, p. xvi)

With the evolution of the brain, symbolic categorization and language allowed the formation of concepts of past and future and models of self and others that were independent of time (Zemke & Clark, 1996). Words, pictures, and ritual acts provided the means for communicating about experiences and feelings and gaining greater control over oneself and one's environment, including changing behavior in ways far beyond the capacity of other species (Csikszentmihalyi & Rochberg-Halton, 1981).

Egypt is credited with giving shape, through religion and hieroglyphics, to mankind's greater awareness of the material and spiritual, natural and cultural duality of the world. From these origins emerged some of the most important and complex symbols that continue to influence contemporary cultures. The zodiac (and the system of destinies represented in its wheel of life), a source of daily guidance for many 20th-century Americans, grew from the study of the planets and their linkage with the gods. Symbols like the triangle, a dominant form in the technology of Egyptian science (i.e., triangulation influenced the study of the rise and fall of rivers and the seasons), appears in the trinity of medieval theology and the philosophy and art of the gothic cathedral; it also represents the smallest unit of procreation (man, woman, and baby) and continues to be evident in religion and all aspects of creativity today (May, 1968).

The efforts currently invested in science and technology were once dedicated to mythology, the "immeasurable wealth of Hindu, Chinese, and Islamic philosophy, the Cabal [Jewish mysticism], and the painstaking investigations of alchemy and similar studies" (Cirlot, 1962, p. xii). The myths of the Mediterranean—expressed in art, legends, and dramatic poetry—conveyed the moral principles, natural laws, and transformations of human life. The tradition of throwing rice, or more environmentally correct birdseed, at newlyweds is a residual of ancient efforts to represent and understand complex human phenomena like fertility through agricultural life. The activities of such classical tragic figures as Hercules, Jason, and Icarus provide timeless lessons about heroics and human struggles with adversity, betrayal, and the risks of over-estimating one's capacities (Henderson, 1964). Today's cult of animated and real-life heroes (Batman, athletes, film stars, and politicians) demonstrates the virtues and vulnerabilities of such figures and the relevance of Greek and Jungian beliefs that the first objective of the hero is to conquer himself (Cirlot, 1962).

The strong traditions that characterized the early symbolist periods were diminished in Western culture from the latter part of the Middle Ages until German romanticism fostered interest in the deeper layers of psychic life as represented in the unconscious and the meanings of dreams (Cirlot, 1962). Before the beginning of this century, Freud and Breuer recognized the symbolic meaning of such conditions as hysteria, certain types of pain, and abnormal behaviors (Jung, 1964). Psychoanalysis and other depth psychologies, the charismatic work of such artists as Chagall and Max Ernst, and the persistent popularity of myths and fairy tales have sustained symbolistic thought through much of the 20th century, although without the vigor that characterized earlier eras of our civilization. While neuroscience, competing psychological theories, and shifts in society's beliefs and values ultimately diminished the status of the psychoanalytic enterprise, symbols and the symbolization process continue to influence us and the activities that define our lives in more ways than many of us imagine.

Commonalities that Transcend Time and Culture

Contemporary tendencies to disassociate from our own inner lives is also reflected in our disengagement from the symbolism of the ancients and primitive cultures. We presume that our advanced reasoning powers, scientific achievements, and education distinguish us at all levels. Archaeologists, anthropologists, and historians have, nonetheless, demonstrated that *the same symbolic patterns* that existed in the myths of the Greeks, the folk stories of American Indians, and the rituals of small tribal societies on the fringe of today's civilization bear relevancy to us as well. If we look closely, we can recognize some of these patterns in the elaborate rituals and symbolic objects associated with such holidays as Christmas and Easter, in our attraction to the heroes of contemporary ticker-tape parades, our devotion to the pomp and circumstance of royal weddings and funerals, and in the strange things we do to bring good luck (crossing our fingers) or ward off evil (spitting over our shoulder three times). The commonalities emerge from the trials and tribulations that are basic to all human existence: in our relationship with ourselves and others, with nature and the universe, and from "traces" left from previous stages of the brain's evolution (Henderson, 1964; Edelman, 1992).

It is this universality of human concerns that became the subject of Jung's concepts of archetypes and the "collective unconscious" (1964). Jung, and Freud before him, proposed the existence of universal symbols that transmit the psychological inheritance of mankind, have deep biological and cultural roots, and reflect struggles about such major life themes as birth, coming of age, the relativity of moral values, and death. For Freud, symbols provided disguises through which repressed internalized conflicts could surface into consciousness, the disguise drawing upon characteristics reminiscent of the body part or process in question. From his perspective, symbolization "transforms the inadmissible into the harmless" (Csikszentmihalyi & Rochberg-Halton, 1981, p. 22) by reducing the tensions associated with unacceptable unconscious wishes. Freud's overdetermined view of human motivation—and the symbolization process—has provoked many theoretical challenges, captured, in part, by his own oft-quoted statement: "Sometimes a cigar is just a cigar" (Bartlett, 1980, p. 679). Ford and Urban vividly state that "one gets the impression that ... adult behavior is ... considered one constant defensive battle, and the creative activities of man are simply by-products, like the trenches and empty cartridges after a real battle" (1963, p. 143). The assumption that all behavior arises from a well of internal instinct-laden energy, interacting with the environment only on the basis of the cues the real world provides, is unreasonable in light of a growing body of knowledge (Fine, 1964).

For Jung (1964), the archetypal instinctual tendencies to form representations of a common motif express needs that extend *beyond* inner conflicts to include powerful desires for personal development and spiritual union with the social and physical environment. His more optimistic approach to human capacity is based "on the transformative potential of symbols ... seen ... as templates for development rather than as simply adjustment" (Csikszentmihalyi & Rochberg-Halton, 1981, p. 25). Jungian archetypes, therefore, tend to focus on the efforts of the self to attain a meaningful balance between individuation and wholeness in the context of society. While representations of these motifs may vary a great deal in detail and bear unique meaning for the individual, they retain their basic patterns. Classic archetypes include such images as heroes and hero makers, the hostile brethren, creation, death and re-birth, whale-dragons, serpents, the moon and sun, good and evil, the damsel in distress, animals, birds, the cosmic fish, and the circle. The emotional energy associated with archetypes can be captured and focused through rituals and other means to move people to action. The ritual repetitions of sacred texts, religious ceremonies, music, and prayers can be used to liberate, comfort, or excite participants. For example, the mandala (the Hindu term for circle), a symbol for achieving order over chaos, appears in Native American sandpaintings where it is used to induce contemplation in tribal healing rituals. It is also the theme of the appealing Streisand (1997) rendition of "Circle,"which speaks to the circle of life and the ways in which diversity and individuality are ultimately balanced by our shared humanity. The same appeal to a group's emotions, however, can be misused to unleash the worst of instincts, as demonstrated by Hitler's use of Teutonic myths to rally German youth to his destructive cause. The reader is directed to Jung's *Man and His Symbols,* Cirlot's *A Dictionary of Symbols,* Caligor and

May's *Dreams and Symbols: Man's Unconscious Language,* and Bettelheim's *The Uses of Enchantment: The Meaning and Importance of Fairy Tales* for a scholarly journey through the collective unconscious.

IN THE ADAPTIVE TRADITION

The search for the meaning of events, actions, emotions and thoughts is one of the great paradoxes of the mind (in so much as) it must use existing models to inter-pret new events; models based on the past must interpret the present and be revised to meet the future. (Horowitz, 1979, p. 242)

The adaptive importance of the symbolization process—the role it plays in connecting those existing "inner life" models with new events, as well as with the collective belief systems of our culture—can be examined from a variety of perspectives. All, however, appear to serve *a transformative function: providing valuable avenues for personal and social differentiation and re-integration.* Put in a more dramatic context—and life's cir-cumstances can be dramatic—one of the most compelling virtues of the symbolization process lies in its contributions to transforming the worst that life has to offer—often turn-ing the dross of adversity into the gold of adaptation and personal accomplishment (Fine, 1991; Vaillant, 1977). How does this happen? The symbolization process mediates con-flicts within the self, represents phenomena not otherwise understood, helps define or express qualities of the self, and binds the social group together—all important elements of coping. In effect, the unconscious "is just as much a vital and real part of the life of an individual as the conscious 'cogitating' world of the ego" (Jung, 1964, p. 12). It is proba-bly more accurate to say that the symbolization process and the unconscious are the unsung partners of the ego. Vaillant's (1993) elegantly crafted *The Wisdom of the Ego* (defined as the integrated and adaptive nervous system) plays out this partnership as he demonstrates the often miraculous ways in which the mind, with all of its inventiveness, helps individuals rise above the particular adversities with which life has presented them. "Think about the irreverent but popular work of cartoonist John Callahan. He has rearranged the ... inner demons of his life (alcoholism at age 11; quadriplegia acquired in an alcohol-related accident) so they are more manageable, purposeful, and acceptable" (Fine, 1993). Each cartoon is, in its own way, a transformative act *providing valuable avenues for personal and social differentiation and re-integration.*

The Individual: Composing a Life

Human development is characterized by an ongoing struggle to both differentiate one-self and belong to the social group. We are on a continuing quest to define and redefine ourselves as the circumstances of our lives change—for better or for worse. Bateson's (1989) artful concept of "composing a life," not unlike Horowitz's comments on the adap-tive process, "... involves a continual reimagining of the future and a reinterpretation of the past to give meaning to the present" (p. 29). As we seek ways to resolve crises of any dimension, the symbolization process (a template for development rather than simply adjustment) provides a means for understanding and managing them, while refining and adding texture to the composition of our lives.

There are many things that defy human understanding, so *we use symbolic terms, images, objects, or actions to represent concepts or experiences that we cannot define or fully comprehend* (Jung, 1964). We see this in the language of a young boy who attempts to explain his or her unpleasant encounter with a cactus by claiming that, "The ouch bit me!" While the boundaries between himself and the inanimate objects around him will assuredly become more differentiated as his cognitive and linguistic capacities mature, the tendency to imbue objects and nature with human traits will continue to serve a purpose as he, and we as adults, try to grasp complex events or social systems. For example, symbolic objects, rituals, and stories serve to distill, simplify, and represent the complex structure and content of religious beliefs. We experience this in the acts and artifacts associated with Holy Communion in which bread and wine are received as a commemoration of the death of Christ. It operates as well during the Passover seder where a roasted shankbone, herbs, horseradish root, haroset, and a roasted egg symbolize ancient sacrifice, hope and renewal, the bitterness of enslavement and forced labor, and the triumph of life over death. Similarly, the symbolic imagery of fairy tales provides manageable means and models for understanding things that might otherwise be beyond one's emotional or cognitive capacity. For the child, stories such as *Hansel and Gretel* or *Cinderella* represent optimistic outcomes of challenging and complex relationships and developmental milestones. Based upon their interests and needs at a given point in time, children may find different meanings in the same story (Bettelheim, 1977).

Symbols also mediate conflicts within the self: *there are many events or possibilities in human experience that are simply too threatening to be easily managed in consciousness in their raw state.* Our mind casts around for ways to experience, understand, and share them. Dreams, and many activities we engage in during our waking hours, serve that purpose. In adult sleep states, for example, anxieties about unpredictable decisions by new office leadership, the fears of an illness, or of one's own fulminating anger may express themselves in a recurring dream in which we are pursued by an aggressive, fiery dragon, until the stressful situation can be manageably formulated in consciousness. Or, consider the dream of a "blocked" writer, preparing an important lecture, who falls into an exhausted sleep only to continue the psychological work of her unfinished paper. In the dream, she is asked to conduct an unfamiliar, large chorus in a lengthy unfamiliar musical composition before an important audience, with no time to rehearse. Filled with fear and trepidation, she raises the baton, and, miraculously, the voices blend together in an inspiring performance. The startled dreamer awakens at the conclusion of her triumph with renewed energy and clarity of purpose and completes her paper within a relatively brief period of time—while humming the music from her dream: the unusual choral finale to Beethoven's "Ninth Symphony," a piece composed (unbeknownst to the dreamer) after a lengthy period of unproductiveness. While interpretations of this dream might take us in many directions, in this situation, the symbolization process most certainly served as a "... great guide, friend, and advisor of the conscious" (Jung, 1964). Whatever else it might mean, its greatest value was in the immediate outcome: renewed focus and confidence, creative problem-solving, and closure.

How one makes sense out of the unusual assemblage of images, storylines, and mixed metaphors in a dream—or any other forms of symbolic expression—is, of course, of importance. Unlike the "musical triumph" of our writer-dreamer, symbolic expressions are usually more puzzling. They are "... not a kind of standardized cryptogram that can be decoded by a glossary of symbol meanings. It is ... a personal expression of the individual, ... a communication that uses symbols common to all mankind, but ... on every occasion in an entirely individual way" (Jung, 1964, p. 13). They may not, however, require formal study and analysis because they may be understood in a subliminal way without interpretation. In former times, people did not reflect upon their symbols. They lived them and were unconsciously animated by their meaning. May (1968) makes a strong case for the inherent intentionality of the unconscious life:

> *The purpose of dreaming is to enable the person to experience rather than explain symbols and myths. Explanations are useful ... only as they open the person up to a fuller experiencing of the (dream). We lose the power of a dream ... when we reduce them to rationalized words, for they then become "signs" rather than "symbols." (p. 9)*

These comments are not intended to diminish the value and importance of seeking appropriate help when symbolization—in dreams, thoughts, or actions—is troubling or one is seeking greater self-understanding. We only need to be wary of oversimplification and stereotypical responses in giving meaning to highly individual symbols.

On a more conscious level, we also use the metaphor or a figure of speech to convey a personal message. Camus' revelation that, "In the depth of winter I finally learned that within me there lay an invincible summer" (as cited by Maquet, 1958) is a vivid example of how a phrase denoting one kind of object or idea (the seasons) is used to convey another (Camus' ability to rise above despair). Individuals confronted with extreme life events (i.e., an illness, incarceration, acts of nature) use the metaphor in poetry and personal narratives to express qualities of the self or to convey what might otherwise be unshareable (Fine, 1991). This is meaningfully demonstrated in the poem of a young boy, whose kinship with trees is inspired by the loss of his own limbs.

When the Tree Falls Down
When the tree falls down
On the ground and
Its heart speeds up
All that's left is
Memories and a very
Pretty cup.

In the cup are
Memories of storms
Times it was almost cut
Down and when it was
Young having fun with
Its parents.

When its cup of
Memories breaks
And its faith cracks
All that's left
Are very beautiful
Naps of thoughts.
—*Adam Jeb* (Berger & Lithwick, 1992, p. 8)

Adam's camp counselor shares some insights derived from having spent much time together:

The beauty of trees is undiminished by their loss of fingers in the fall or limbs in storms. Trees cannot move like the other creatures, but that is why they are able to hold so much life and song. The trees in Adam's poems hold the burden of his memories, while his 8-year-old imagination climbs into their highest branches. (p. 3)

For both Camus and Adam, the metaphor resonates with the reader and seems to empower these personal experiences in ways more literal language never could.

The Collective Beliefs of Culture

The original meaning of the symbol—that which brings people together—continues to be its most highly valued feature. If we return to Read's quote about the increased need for symbolism as industrialization has altered man's life, we understand more fully the complexities and contradictions inherent in striving to both achieve individuation and maintain collective belief systems. Whether an outgrowth of market specialization and competitiveness, urbanization, developments in modern science, or what critic Robert Hughes (1993) refers to as a weakened politics of ideology, "the traditional American genius for consensus, for getting along by making up practical compromises to meet real social needs" (p.13) has been diminished, and with it the sense of collectivity that has defined this country. However, concerns about the deterioration of society are not unique to this era of social commentary. At the turn of the century, concerns about the decline and fragmentation of Western society led Freud, Jung, Durkeim, Simmel, and others to examine "the ways meaning is created and how it serves to bind society together" (Csikszentmihalyi & Rochberg-Halton, 1981, p. 41).

For those immersed in the psychological world of the individual, the imposing impact of culture is often forgotten. Bruner reminds us that the

morphological steps in evolution ... would not have mattered save for the concurrent emergence of shared symbolic systems, of traditionalized ways of living and working together—in short, of human culture. They constitute a very special kind of communal tool kit whose tools, once used, (make) the user a reflection of the community. (1990, p. 11)

Folk Psychology and Narratives

Some of those tools—narratives, fairy tales, and rituals—are part of what Bruner refers to as *folk psychology ... a culture's account of what makes human beings tick* (1990, p. 14). Folk psychology speaks to ways people anticipate and judge one another, draw conclusions about the meaningfulness of their lives, determine how they will commit themselves to particular modes of life. "Its power over human mental function and human life is that it provides the very means by which culture shapes human beings to its requirements" (p. 15). Its organizing principles are *narrative* and not conceptual.

The "art of the narrative" has acquired greater visibility in the past decade. Bateson believes that "storytelling is fundamental to the human search for meaning whether we tell tales of the creation of the earth or of our own early choices" (1990, p. 34). The reader is referred to Kleinman's *The Illness Narratives: Suffering, Healing, and the Human*

Condition, Langness and Frank's *Lives: An Anthropological Approach to Biography*, and to Bruner's *Acts of Meaning*. While broadening our understanding of cultures (including the social context of illness), they also provide a vivid contemporary counterpoint to and explanation of the role of traditional folk and fairy tales. They help us to understand the values, mission, milestones, and everyday activities of a culture and the place the individual makes for himself or herself within that social group. And, ultimately, the particular symbolic themes, forms, and objects that are apt to acquire the most meaning. The author is reminded of the woman, hospitalized following a stroke, who kept worrying about her children's laundry, although this and other household chores were being effectively managed by others. As her personal narrative emerged, it became clear that she, like Bateson (1990), "found special satisfaction (in) repetitive tasks that have an underlying, barely perceptible rhythm of change, such as washing and folding blue jeans that grow gradually larger over the course of a childhood" (p. 213)—and she was at great risk for not being able to engage in that housewifely ritual—or live long enough to watch those jeans change over time (Fine, 1993).

The special meaning of laundry—the alleged albatross on the backs of many women— is a striking example of the complex ways in which *the nonhuman environment and objects are dynamic—but often neglected—factors in our lives.* Searles (1960) and Csikszentmihalyi and Rochberg-Halton (1981) provide a challenging and convincing dialectic about the ways in which objects fill our lives and influence our behavior throughout the life cycle. We need only examine our own object histories to appreciate the multi-layered meaning of a beloved family pet, the carefully catalogued baseball cards of our childhood, a locket handed down from grandmother to granddaughter, a treasured copy of Kahlil Gibran's *The Prophet*, an adult's weekend schoolyard pick-up basketball game, or singular devotion to the care and nurturing of his or her automobile.

Rituals and Performance

Turner's (1988) decades of work on the structure and meaning of ritual and performance provide valuable insights into the way symbolic images, objects, and activities influence the growth and change of a culture. He sees rituals as the performance of a complex sequence of symbolic acts and transformative efforts to manage social dramas or personal crises that contradict or challenge social processes that may erupt, for example, when someone, legitimately or illegitimately, begins to move to a new position in the social order. This change may be facilitated, or obstructed, through ritualized or ceremonial methods that serve to reorganize and legitimize the social structure. We are familiar with many of the ancient and contemporary rituals used for birth, initiation/rites of passage, marriage, and death. In each of these, change and potential crises are transformed into occasions where symbols and values representing unity and continuity of the group are celebrated. The large, festive, and long-lasting ritual wedding ceremonies of orthodox Judaism and Indian cultures are excellent examples. Turner purports that "... ritual is not necessarily a bastion of social conservatism; its symbols do not merely condense cherished sociocultural values. Rather, through its liminal processes, it holds the generating source of culture and structure" (1988, p. 11). Turner's use of the term liminal, "the betwixt and between, a threshold," captures the notion of a dynamic, rather than fixed process that links "performative behavior: art, sports, ritual, play with social and ethical structure—or—the way people think about and organize their lives and specify individual and group values" (p. 8).

Believing that "all performance has at its core a ritual action, a restoration of behavior" (p. 7), Turner promotes performance as intending to both express and critique the culture it is part of through a complex sequence of symbolic acts. His discussion of the very colorful, annual *Brazilian Carnaval* demonstrates the ways in which a country expresses its "subjective mood, ... its mood of feeling, willing and desiring, its mood of fantasizing, its playful mood" (p. 123)—as opposed to its usual effort to apply reason to human action. The masks and costumes, music and dancing, feasting and drinking that induces disequilibrium and alters reality and consciousness are intended to turn cultural values upside down and examine them in many forms and modalities.

Ritual dramas and other performance genres (i.e., Japanese Noh or Kabuki theatre) are often multimedia orchestrations, conducted by a master of ceremonies (i.e., *Cabaret*), storyteller (i.e., *The Lion King*), choreographer (i.e., *Chorus Line*), or priest, that may involve distinctive aromas, visual cues, gestures, sounds, and facial expressions that have been assigned different meanings. "Their full meaning emerges from the union of script with actors and audience at a given moment in a group's ongoing social process" (p. 24).

Turner's study of *performance art as process* casts a special light on the value of the working experience before, as well as during, the formal presentation. Rehearsals for shows, team practice for athletic events, and the highly organized year-long preparation of costumes and Samba competitions for *Carnaval* bring participants together in dynamic ways that influence and alter social processes and convey a new awareness or perspective about individual and cultural beliefs and concerns.

Disney's film *Fantasia* represents such a contemporary American phenomena. As the first multimedia extravaganza of its kind, integrating classical music, a wide screen, dimensional sound, and innovative animation techniques, Disney provided the public with a multisensory performance genre that has sustained its charismatic impact for decades. The power of *Fantasia* is in the remembering, as evidenced by the expressiveness of adults telling of their first and often repeated experiences with this film. They have not forgotten the terror of *The Night on Bald Mountain*, the delight of thistles and orchids transformed into dancing Cossacks and peasant girls, the touching familiarity of Hop-Lo's out-of-synch experiences, and the mythic nature of flying horses and centaurs. These motifs stay with us because their appeal extends beyond aesthetic art to a transformative experience. The stories address social dramas and personal crises: "the ... despair a dinosaur shows when it knows it is going to die; how the smallest mushroom in a group moves when he is trying to get in step; how the God of Evil reacts when he realizes that the power of good is too strong for him" (Culhane, 1983, p. 28). In *Fantasia*, the apprentice, usurping the sorcerer's power, sets in motion forces beyond his control. And, just as Disney's *Who's Afraid of the Big Bad Wolf* of the 1930s served as folklore for the Great Depression, this story has become folklore for the Nuclear Age.

The performance experience for the audience is only one dimension of the meaning-making power of this film. Consider the creative and social group process that emerged during the 3-year production of the film. The story conference method that characterized the Disney approach generated hundreds of pages of stenographic notes, much like an anthropologist's ethnographic studies. They documented the birth and evolution of ideas, stories, and characters and the interaction among animators, story developers, musicians, technicians, and Disney himself. Reaching into their own psychic reservoirs, they sought to "make a rich, colorful, complicated story of great philosophic importance in six or seven simple little happy sequences with a mixture of awesome fantasy and great comedy" (p. 24). The experience, according to animator Bill Tytla, was akin to "feeling that you're going to grab that goddam Holy Grail" (p. 20). There are those who believe they did!

Fantasia, like *Carnaval* and many other performance experiences, uses the creative language of symbolic image and action to depict, explore, and change the ways we think about and organize our lives and our beliefs. As tools used in the service of personal and societal adaptation, they ingeniously demonstrate how activities at one level influence processes at another.

CONCLUSION

If we turn once more to Bettelheim's belief that living in true consciousness requires finding meaning in our lives, we must acknowledge the curious ways in which consciousness draws upon that which is not conscious. This chapter, and the book of which it is a part, challenge the reader to examine the symbolization process as a tool of meaning; a bridge and inventive intermediary between man's inner life and external reality. It also asks the reader to suspend pre-existing beliefs and biases and reflect upon the purpose and processes that define symbolization. Symbol formation—the conscious representation of unconscious mental content—is an extraordinary mechanism by which we communicate with ourselves and others. While it may take the form of disruptive emotional and physical symptoms at times, it is also a process by which creative and constructive events unfold daily. The mysterious nature of this process—neuroscience aside—has a tenacious hold on the history and the "here-and-now" of civilization. Our rational selves and our cultures are greatly enriched by symbolic language, image, and ritual.

In revisiting the existential dilemma of how we find and give meaning to our lives, one is inevitably drawn to Vaillant's *Adaptation to Life* (1977). The spirit and substance of his inquiry into the differentiated hierarchy of ego functions tells the story of how symbolic transformations generate healthy adaptation in those who have had to overcome enormous barriers. He reminds us that

> *our task as members of ... society is to take pains that our culture and or own behavior enable others to play games, to achieve art, to enjoy their work. We must ask ourselves how we can help a paranoid's projection become a novel, an eccentric's sexual fantasy become a sculpture, and a delinquent's impulse to murder evolve into creative law-making or into the subtleties of a New Yorker cartoon.*

These transformations occur on a daily basis and under much less dramatic circumstances as well. The process—peculiar to each, yet shared by many—is an astonishing product of the integrated capacity of the mind, brain, and culture to create and give meaning to life.

REFERENCES

Bartlett, J. (1980). *Bartlett's familiar quotations.* Boston: Little, Brown, and Company.

Bateson, M. C. (1990). *Composing a life.* New York: Plume Books.

Berger, L., & Lithwick, D. (1992). *I will sing life: Voices from the Hole in the Wall Gang camp.* Boston: Little, Brown and Co.

Bettelheim, B. (1977). *The uses of enchantment: The meaning and importance of fairy tales.* New York: Alfred A. Knopf.

Bruner, J. (1990). *Acts of meaning.* Cambridge, Mass: Harvard University Press.

Cirlot, J. E. (1962). *A dictionary of symbols.* New York: Philosophical Library.

Csikszentmihalyi, M., & Rochberg-Halton, E. (1981). *The meaning of things: Domestic symbols and the self.* New York: Cambridge University Press.

Culhane, J. (1983). *Walt Disney's Fantasia.* New York: Harry N. Abrams, Inc.

Edelman, G. M. (1992). *Bright air, brilliant fire.* New York: Basic Books.

Fine, S. B. (1964). *The analytic model: Behavior is more than it appears to be.* Presentation at The World Federation of Occupational Therapy, Jerusalem.

Fine, S. B. (1991). Resilience and human adaptability: Who rises above adversity. Eleanor Clarke Slagle Lecture. *Am J Occup Ther, 45,* 493-503.

Fine, S. B. (1993). Interaction between psychosocial variables and cognitive function. In: C. B. Royeen (Ed.). *AOTA self study series: Cognitive rehabilitation.* Rockville, MD: American Occupational Therapy Association.

Ford, D. H., & Urban, H. (1963). *Systems of psychotherapy.* New York: Wiley & Sons, Inc.

Freud, S. (1955). *The interpretation of dreams.* New York: Basic Books.

Gazzaniga, M. S. (1988). *Mind matters: How the mind & brain interact to create our conscious lives.* Boston: Houghton Mifflin Company.

Henderson, J. L. (1964). Ancient myths and modern man. In: C. Jung (Ed.). *Man and his symbols.* London: Aldus Books Limited.

Horowitz, M. J. (1979). Psychological response to serious life events. In: V. Hamilton & D. M. Warburton (Eds.). *Human stress and cognition* (pp. 237-263). New York: Wiley.

Hughes, R. (1993). *Culture of complaint: The fraying of America.* New York: Oxford University Press.

Jung, C. G. (1964). *Man and his symbols.* London: Aldus Books Limited.

Kleinman, A. (1988). *The illness narratives: Suffering, healing and the human condition.* New York: Basic Books.

Konner, M. (1982). *The tangled wing.* New York: Holt, Rinehart & Winston.

Langness, L. L., & Frank, G. (1986). *Lives: An anthropological approach to biography.* Novato, CA: Chandler & Sharp Publishers.

Lazarus, R. S., & Folkman, S. (1984). *Stress, appraisal and coping.* New York: Springer.

Maquet, A. (1958). *Albert Camus: The invincible summer.* New York: Braziller.

May, R. (1968): Part I: Dreams and symbols. In: L. Caligor & R. May. *Dreams and symbols.* New York: Basic Books, Inc.

Paz, O. (1998). Untitled poem. In: *New York Times,* April 25.

Read, H. (1962). Forward. In: J. E. Cirlot, *A dictionary of symbols.* New York: Philosophical Library.

Sacks, O. (1964). *A leg to stand on.* New York: Harper & Row.

Searles, H. F. (1960). *The nonhuman environment.* New York: International University Press.

Streisand, B. (1997). Circle. In *Higher Ground.* New York: Columbia Records.

Turner, V. (1988). *The anthropology of performance.* New York: PAJ Publications.

Vaillant, G. E. (1977). *Adaptation to life.* Boston, Mass: Little, Brown, and Co. Limited.

Vaillant, G. E. (1993). *The wisdom of the ego.* Cambridge, Mass: Harvard University Press.

Zemke, R., & Clark, F. (1996). *Occupational science: The evolving discipline.* Philadelphia: F. A. Davis Co.

ADDITIONAL READING

Arieti, S. (1976). *Creativity: The magic synthesis.* New York: Basic Books.

Bulfinch, T. (1966). *Bulfinch's mythology.* London: Spring Books.

Coles, R. (1990). *The spiritual life of children.* Boston: Houghton Mifflin Co.

Graves, R., & Patal, R. (1983). *Hebrew myths: The Book of Genesis.* New York: Greenwich House.

Gregory, R. L. (1987). *The Oxford companion to the mind.* Oxford, England: Oxford University Press.

Jaffe, A. (1964). Symbolism in the visual arts. In: C. Jung (Ed.). *Man and his symbols.* London: Aldus Books Limited.

Kris, E. (1952). *Psychoanalytic explorations in art.* New York: International Universities Press, Inc.

Langer, S. (1956). *Philosophy in a new key—A study in the symbolism of reason, rite and art.* New York: Mentor Books.

Leymarie, J. (1967). *Marc Chagall: The Jerusalem windows.* New York: George Braziller.

Meyer, F. (1957). *Marc Chagall: Life and work.* New York: Harry N. Abrams, Inc.

Polkinghorne, D. (1988). Narrative knowing and the human sciences.

Exploring Potential: The Activity Laboratory

Gail S. Fidler

The speculation that "every human expression means more than it seems" (Erikson, 1976, p. 41) rings truer as the world of symbols and metaphors is explored. This is especially so as the richly varied characteristics and textures of activities, the statements they make, and the related responses they evoke begin to emerge. Each subsequent chapter in this text offers a special focus and dimension of this pursuit. However, experience has shown that, when a series of carefully planned activity experiences precede such study and when each is immediately followed by guided reflection and critique, learning is accelerated and a heightened level of readiness for continued exploration is reached.

This specially designed, experiential introduction should engage the learner as participant in activities that are chosen to provide a microcosm of the processes and content of subsequent study. This planned learning is intended to do the following:

- Tease out a beginning awareness that there is more to an activity than meets the eye, more than what is manifest.
- Begin recognition of the significance of the multidimensional characteristics of an activity and of how parts inter-relate to form the whole.
- Nurture an increasing comfort with the abstract, with exploring and questioning symbolic inferences, metaphors, and meanings in everyday activities.
- Encourage and provide practice in applying the critical, analytical, and reflective processes of reasoning to the study of activities.

- Stimulate and support a healthy respect for self and one's own experiences as a valuable teacher and resource.
- Introduce the process of comparative analysis of qualitative procedure as the preferred method for assessing and describing the nature of an activity.
- Generate a beginning suspicion that an activity does indeed have meaning in and of itself.
- Formulate a number of questions from which to further examine, critique, and question the inherent meanings of activities.

Several important factors must be taken into account in the design of the content-focus, the procedures and environmental context of an introductory activity laboratory. Each activity selected should be chosen because it clearly and unambiguously represents a certain category or class of activities, such as, for example, an activity that clearly represents a high degree of structure or one with outstanding characteristics of competition or interpersonal strategy.

To emphasize the process of comparative analysis in describing and assessing activities, those chosen for this laboratory experience should be markedly different, clearly in contrast with one another. When, for instance, a highly structured activity devoid of ambiguity is followed by one without evident structure, or a solitary activity precedes one requiring strategy and collaboration, the comparative process in assessment becomes evident, and the unique characteristics of each are emphasized.

Because of the value of the accumulation of experiences, of the immediate carry-over of what has just been discovered or learned to a new experience, the planned sequence of carefully selected activities should be offered within a single block of time. The number of activities within this timeframe should be limited to reduce the risk of overload. Furthermore, each activity should be able to be completed and thoroughly discussed within a 60-minute block of time. Four activities within a single 4-hour timeframe have proven to be a very satisfactory format.

As each activity is completed, an open discussion of the experience should immediately follow. It is important that critique of the activity experience be centered on the activity, not the performer. All responses, observations, and inferences should always be examined in terms of which elements of the activity seem to have elicited the response and how the impact of the activity can be explained in relation to the nature of the activity. Participants' reactions are significant because they demonstrate ways in which an activity, by the nature of its characteristics, can evoke certain thoughts, feelings, and behaviors. However, the laboratory is not a projective technique. Its purpose is to gain an understanding of the nature of the activity, not the person. Some questions that will stimulate dialogue and will serve to maintain focus at the conclusion of each activity include the following:

- What did you like about this activity? How do your reactions relate to the objects or materials of the activity, to its procedures and rules, to its action requirements? What sociocultural meanings do these suggest to you?
- What did you not like about this activity? The previous questions should be raised in relation to this question.
- What was the most difficult experience to manage? How do these responses relate to the elements of properties, structure, action processes, and sociocultural meanings?
- What responses were triggered by this activity that were not evident in previous ones? How are the activities different?
- What activities from your daily experiences are similar to this activity? How are they

alike? What activities have you experienced that are very different? What makes them very different from this activity?

- What symbols or intended meanings were you aware of?

Consensual validation, the agreement on the nature of "the thing," is an important construct in the investigation of the nature and meaning of an activity. The question of how many others share one's point of view or have similar ideas and reactions is significant in gaining some perspective on the validity of suppositions. It is, therefore, useful to look at the extent of agreement and differences throughout the discussion.

The Activity Laboratory was originally designed in 1965 as a teaching and diagnostic procedure. It was later published as a process for observing and assessing perceptual and behavioral strategies (Fidler, 1982). For more than 30 years, this laboratory has been used as a teaching-learning experience for thousands of students and interdisciplinary professionals throughout the United States. Its broad use over these many years with both client and professional groups has made it possible to compare responses, clarify differences in the characteristics and sociocultural significance of activities, demonstrate agreement on the nature of these characteristics, and consensually validate the thesis that an activity does indeed have a "character," a language of its own. (The following material has been adapted from Fidler, 1982.)

As a teaching-learning process, the laboratory comprises four activities, offered in sequence and within a single 4-hour time frame. The four activities include a cut-out and crayon project, a finger painting, a collage, and a circle ball tag game. These were chosen because they best met the criteria for such a laboratory. However, these can be replaced by other activities as long as the criteria for choice is met.

The first activity offered is a cut-out and crayon project. Two drawings (Figures 3-1a and 3-1b), each centered on an 8½" x 5½" sheet of white bond paper, are provided along with a sheet of 8½" x 11" white bond paper, one pair of small scissors, and two crayons, one dark color and one light color.

The participant is asked to choose one of the two drawings, cut out the drawing, retrace it on the blank sheet of paper, and then color in the form and background, using the light color for background and the dark color for the form. To reinforce structure and external control, it is very important that the laboratory setting be prepared and set up in accordance with the following instructions before the students arrive. Both drawings are placed evenly on top of one another and then on top of the blank paper. These are placed vertically on the table in the center of each seating arrangement. The small pair of scissors and the dark and light crayons are placed horizontally at the top center of the papers. The time limit is 30 minutes.

At its completion, the students are asked to critique and discuss their responses to the experience. Free discussion should be encouraged and guided in part by the questions mentioned earlier. The responsibility of the instructor is to guide rather than lead this process, while maintaining the participants' focus on identifying and describing the salient characteristics of the activity and the responses they elicited. To guide this focus, it is important for the instructor to keep the following in mind.

Cut-Out and Crayon Activity

The cut-out and crayon activity is one that realistically and symbolically contains a high degree of external limits and controls. Outcome expectations are clear and pre-

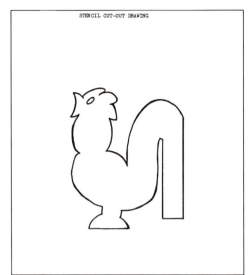
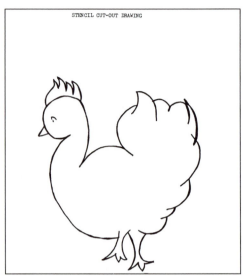

Figures 3-1a and 3-1b. The first activity in the Activity Laboratory requires the participant to choose one of two drawings (as above), cut it out with scissors, retrace it on a blank sheet of paper, then color in the form and background.

dictable, and processes are sequentially ordered and controlled by pattern, materials, and directions. The only explicitly free choice is the instruction to select one of the two forms for reproduction. The nature of the task, the structure of the setting in which it occurs, and the materials used are most reminiscent of early school years and of child-to-authority relationships.

The activity requires a moderate degree of fine motor skills. The social-interpersonal field requires no interdependent collaborative behavior. It is one of parallel activity with implied expectations that each participant function independently without influence on or from another. The two figures of choice present quite contrasting orientations: one a stylized, stationary, solid-looking, crowing creature; the other, a softer looking, fluffy, more fluid and intricately drawn creature.

This activity will, because of its characteristics, most readily evoke response about styles and patterns of responding to and managing clearly established external limits and controls, cause and effect predictability, sequential ordering, restrictions on free choice and individuality, risk taking and chance, inferred limitations and task expectations, and moderately fine motor skill requirements. Responses to the two figures are most frequently related to the symbolic statements they make. Responses to the perceived difficulty or ease of cutting out one or the other forms are not infrequent.

FINGER PAINTING

Finger painting is the second activity offered. Large finger-painting paper, approximately 24 inches x 18 inches, is provided. Red, blue, green, yellow, black, and brown colors are placed along the center of the table. Containers of water are placed around the table. This activity is offered without structure, and the participants are asked to simply take a piece of paper and work with the paints on that paper. When each participant has completed the assignment or when the 30-minute time limit has been reached, a discussion about the activity takes place following the same format as previously mentioned.

This is an activity that realistically and symbolically contains a high degree of freedom in terms of process and outcomes. External limits and controls are virtually non-existent, except in an inferred manner by the size of the paper. There are no rules or patterns to govern process, control decisions, define outcomes, or act as an organizing, task initiating force. Freedom from external limits and control is reinforced by the fluid nature of the paint and water and the smooth surface of the paper. These support the quality of unpredictability and the element of chance. The lack of structure, coupled with the fluid nature of the materials and the direct hand contact with the paint, establishes the self as the initiator—the cause and effect agent. Color, texture, smell, and hand-arm movement with the paint are sensory and affective stimuli that restate the free, self-expressive nature of the activity. Permanency of an end product is a matter of free choice. Finger painting is most frequently associated with childhood experiences, free expression, and play.

There are no fine motor skill requirements. The social-interpersonal field does not require interdependent, collaborative behavior.

Because of these characteristics, this activity will most readily elicit responses about styles and manners of responding to and managing unstructured tasks and settings; freedom from external controls and limits; risk, chanciness, and change; sensory and affective stimuli; expectations regarding self-expression, initiative, individuality, and spontaneity.

COLLAGE

The third activity offered is a *collage*. Large sheets (approximately 24" x 18") of various colors of construction paper are provided, along with several containers of glue or paste, scissors, and a large and varied assortment of materials and objects to include such items as buttons, fabric, straws, ribbon, string, cotton, cards, etc. It is important that materials and objects for the collage be as varied and in as large a quantity as possible. The variety of both stimuli and options is a critical factor. The materials should be placed on a table other than the one used for working. Participants are asked to select a large sheet of colored construction paper, choose any material from the table, and arrange these in any way they please on the paper to form an abstract picture, to convey a thought or idea.

This activity requires a moderate degree of cognitive organization. The numerous and varied materials and objects available for use and the specifications for the end product comprise a task that requires organization of sensory stimuli and thought. External organizing factors, such as a pattern, guidelines, or directions, are absent. The process involves perceiving the number of possible alternatives, such as what resources are available and what end product might be possible; assessing the applicability of resources (objects, materials, personal skills, and time) in relation to outcome plan; making a choice; organizing and planning in accordance with that choice; adapting, altering, and reassessing the plan and materials; following through and implementing the plan; being goal directed; and inhibiting other alternatives and stimuli that are extraneous or counter-productive to the chosen plan. Volition is, thus, a critical element, as is judgment.

The materials and objects used all have a history and, thus, a consensually validated use and purpose in everyday life, such as buttons, twine, fabric, ads, and greeting cards. The activity requires a degree of abstraction, the envisioning and use of materials and objects out of context of their traditional uses or purposes. Interpersonal skills are required only to the degree of being able to share scissors, glue, and the common stockpile of materials. It is a parallel activity with the implied expectation of independence without influence on or from others. No significant degree of fine motor skills is required. A moderate ability to manage spatial relationships and three-dimensional perspectives is necessary.

This activity will, therefore, most usually evoke responses related to styles and patterns of responding to and/or managing multiple, varied, and simultaneous sensory and ideational stimuli; sequential problem-solving processes that involve identifying options, assessing alternatives, organizing, and planning without external structure for the process or end product achievement; reassessing, altering, and compromising ideas and plans; implementing and following through on a self-designed plan; organization, initiation, abstraction, and reality testing; time management; and interpersonal and social expectations inherent in such a task and environment.

CIRCLE BALL TAG

The fourth and final activity of the laboratory consists of a game of *circle ball tag*. A circle is formed, and one person volunteers or is chosen to be in the center of the circle. Those in the circle throw the ball across the circle, and the person in the center is expected to intercept and catch the ball. When the ball is caught, the person who has thrown the ball must move into the center of the circle. The game is played until all persons have had at least one opportunity to be in the center of the circle.

This activity requires a moderate degree of gross motor coordination and physical assertion. The game is one of competition and cooperative play. It requires attentiveness to the behavior and activity of others, anticipation and judgment about the movement of another, motor planning, and execution. Competition involves the one-against-one and group-against-one, and a test of gross motor planning and agility. The structure, process, and purpose of the game allows for individual choice of one-to-one and/or an alliance with others to compete against or help the person in the center of the circle. In this context, alteration of the basic ground rules is neither prohibited nor explicitly expected. The development of a consensus with regard to helping out or making it more difficult for the one in the center position requires initiating behavior, responding to cues from others, and an incentive to join one or another alliance. The center of the circle position involves coordination of the body in movement, physical assertiveness, second-guessing others, motor planning, agility, and competitiveness.

This activity will, therefore, evoke responses related to styles and patterns of responding to and/or managing gross motor skills; balance, control, and coordination in movement; physical assertion energy and forcefulness; motor planning, alertness, and agility; competition, success, failure, and frustration; cooperative, responsive expectations; the skills, limitations, and feelings of others; scapegoat, aggressor, mediator, or helper roles; group identification; and collaborative expectations.

The Activity Laboratory is a unique experience for most students and many experienced professionals. It reaffirms that a participatory experience that is thoughtfully planned can become a remarkable teacher. This laboratory experience enables exploration of how highly structured activities with clear rules and procedures evoke associations and behaviors that relate to coping with and managing external limits, of putting the puzzle together. By contrast, one is able to see how activities with limited or no structure can, through their creative elements, elicit responses related to managing freedom and lack of external control and direction. The laboratory, furthermore, makes it possible to experience ways in which the performance requirements of an activity for decision making, organization, judgment, or interpersonal strategies and competitive behavior trigger relevant responses.

The laboratory offers experiences in which the learners can attend to the here and now happenings, associate these with their daily life activity experiences, and reflect on and critique this "joining" at their own pace and level of learning readiness. It is a beginning point of coming to see how the objective reality, the symbolic, and the subjective come together to create a dynamic whole; to begin to appreciate that every activity is indeed more than it seems; and to be challenged to a more substantive study and discovery (Fidler, 1982).

REFERENCES

Erikson, E. (1976). *Toys and reason, stages in the ritualization of experience.* New York: W. W. Norton.

Fidler G. S. (1982). The activity laboratory: A structure for observing and assessing perceptual, integrative, and behavioral strategies. In: B. Hemphill (Ed.), *The evaluative process in psychiatric occupational therapy.* Thorofare, NJ: SLACK Incorporated.

Read H. (1958). *Education through art.* London: Farber and Farber.

The Language of Objects

Gail S. Fidler

Engagement with objects is ubiquitous throughout our everyday life. The computer, television, boom box, cellular phone, dishwasher, and clothes dryer, for example, are indisputable objects of our culture. Each has an explicit function, each has sociocultural meanings, and each triggers idiosyncratic, subjective responses. Objects are dynamic entities integrally linked with action. Their meaning is derived through the activity associated with them and in the end goal of the interaction. The special toys and associated activities of childhood, the treasured objects of adolescence, and the object relationships that characterize adulthood and aging weave a lifetime story of self and relatedness to one's world.

In support of this thesis, Csikszentmihalyi and Rochberg-Halton (1981) contended that to "understand what people are and what they might become, one must understand what goes on between people and things" (p. 1). This chapter is devoted to looking at some of what goes on between people and "things." The role of objects, the nature and quality of transactions with them, and the relevance of such involvement in shaping individual attitudes, values, and interpersonal skills will be explored. This undertaking should build a foundation for subsequent study and exploration of the characteristics of various activities and the dynamics of engagement.

The Object History (Fine & Fidler, 1971) was developed to provide a guideline for reflection and the subsequent recording of an individual's attachment to and engagement with those objects that held special, personal meaning. Objects are an important part of activities. Understanding their meaning and role in shaping attitudes and behaviors is critical for understanding and coming to value the many dimensions of activities. The process of reflecting on and recording one's own involvement with objects brings into awareness the significance of these engagements in one's timely motor, perceptual, cognitive, and affective development. Similarly, the role of object relationships in addressing personal issues, concerns, fears, and interests becomes increasingly clear.

OBJECT HISTORY

An object history is a descriptive account of the ways in which certain nonhuman objects (animate and inanimate) are significantly linked with phases of an individual's growth and development.

Please select an object that had special meaning to you during the early years of your life. Use your recollections as well as those of your family. Photo albums and attics help too. Objects may range from toys, animals, household items, objects of nature, clothing, food, etc.—any nonhuman object.

Record the following in your object history:
1. Describe the objects, its name, physical properties, and outstanding characteristics.
2. Identify the source of the object (gift, self-discovered, received from a special person, etc.).
3. Describe how you played with, used, and/or were involved with the object.
4. Describe what seems to have been the meaning and importance of the object to you in terms of your emotional, social, intellectual, and physical development at that time.
5. Describe how members of your family and friends were aware of or involved with your object.
6. How was your relationship with the object ended?
7. How are your treasured objects of today similar to and different from this earlier object?

Sharing and comparing one's own object history with peers offers a unique opportunity for validating meanings and exploring personal and sociocultural differences and similarities. These dialogues facilitate the discovery and examination of personal and cultural differences in both the choice and use of objects and the varying social roles, values, and behaviors that are learned, reinforced, and reflected through objects and their related activity. Experience over time has validated the richness of the learning that derives from these processes for both learner and teacher.

Having children tell stories built around a treasured toy or a particular object from a favorite game contributes significantly to learning about the role and meaning of the object. Additionally, it is a thoroughly enjoyable and rewarding experience for both the child and the adult who engages the child in this activity. Developing an object history with residents in nursing homes and senior citizen centers and having them share these in small peer groups provides noteworthy learning about objects and activities and is a remarkable self-validating experience for the older adult.

More than 30 years ago, Searles (1960) published his study of the nonhuman environment. These investigations indicated that engagement with nonhuman objects (animate and inanimate) was a significant force in the development of human thought and behavior. The concepts he developed from this study have continued to hold validity and relevance to this day. The following adaptations represent a number of these concepts as they relate to the role of nonhuman objects in human growth and development. As these are discussed, additional examples from the learner's experience should be elicited to further illustrate each point.

- *Developing a sense of self as a human:* Coming to know ones self as a human is an ongoing process throughout life. It requires living with humans, as well as engaging with one's nonhuman world. It involves the ongoing process of differentiating self from nonhuman objects, discerning the animate and human from animate and nonhuman, and distinguishing actions and events related to human endeavor from nonhuman or the activity of nature. Involvement with a pet, the contrasting inertness of the teddy bear, and meeting the challenges of the two-wheeler, skis, chessboard, or mountain top are only a few examples of learning to discern animate from inanimate, human from nonhuman, and the nature of self. Each of the following attributes of object relationships contribute to the sense of being human as well as to the sense of self.

- *Becoming aware of feelings and of one's capacity for feeling:* Coming to know one's feelings through fondness for a toy, winning or losing a game, coping with a difficult task, participating in a team sport, and reading sad, funny, or scary stories are important experiences in developing the capacity to feel and in increasing one's comfort and awareness of emotions.

- *Learning how to manage emotions:* Confronting the challenge of a competitive sport, nurturing and training a pet, managing the canoe or sailboat, playing a musical instrument, or racing a horse are a few examples of involvement with objects that help us learn to be sensitive managers of self.

- *Perceiving feelings in others:* Observing how others handle and relate to their object world offers important dimensions to understanding self and others. How parents, siblings, and other significant people engage with a pet, relate to special objects, behave in an activity, and respond to or value the activity of others provides a context from which expectations and predictions about the values and behaviors of others can evolve. The popularity of spectator sports and television dramas is evidence of how important this process is in understanding and coping with one's world and of knowing, differentiating, and relating self to that world.

- *Expressing and coping with conflict, fears, and doubts:* Play acting; disciplining the doll; engaging the toy soldiers, the spacemen, or the puppet; writing a poem; producing a play; engaging in strenuous physical activity; trying out a new venture; and taking a walk are examples of the tried and true ways each of us use to express and explore ways of coping with and of working out our conflicts, doubts, and fears.

- *Practice in the development of skills:* Engagement with nonhuman objects and the activities associated with these is a rich source for exploring abilities and trying out and practicing what one can do. Testing and challenging one's skill in handling the ball, managing the in-line skates or the computer, constructing the bird house, repairing the faucet, or managing the latch hook are all parts of discovering, testing, and developing one's skills of doing.

- *Responding to and satisfying interests and needs:* Exploring and discovering interests, finding ways of being responsive to one's own needs through, for example, loving and caring for a pet, a special object or toy, planting a garden, painting a picture, playing or listening to music, being a cause, constructing, making things happen. These experiences represent critical aspects of becoming, of evolving an identity, a sense of self as having worthy, acceptable needs and desires, and of being able to actualize these.

- *Experimenting with ways of relating and communicating:* The internalized sense of self as an acceptable, valuable human being evolves in part out of and in turn is reflected in one's communication skills and patterns. Sharing activity experiences with others, creating and giving objects to others, being involved in activities that contribute to the welfare of others, being a team member, and working with habitat are only a few examples of how engagement with objects and their related activity provide opportunities to experiment with ways of relating, connecting, and communicating.

More recently, Csikszentmihalyi and Rochberg-Halton (1981) have made an impressive contribution toward understanding the meaning and role of objects in the lives of individuals, in shaping and reflecting cultures, and in recording history. These scientists studied the meaning of household objects in the lives of several hundred people. What they have produced goes a long way toward validating the hypotheses that objects and activity are intimately related; that objects have practical as well as symbolic, subjective meaning, a duality of reality and metaphor; and that objects and their associated activity significantly influence and define the self and one's sociocultural world.

Although much of the material that follows in this chapter relies heavily on the study of these researchers, the following material cannot replace their published work (1981) as an essential resource for studying object relationships.

Objects are considered signs, in the sense of the reality of their meaning. They are viewed as reflecting and shaping the owner, thus creating the person as well as the person giving meaning to the object. It is contended that, because they do not exist in the abstract, people are what they attend to, cherish, use, and make. Objects and our engagement with them are inseparable from who we are, and these relationships actually change how we view ourselves. The degree of similarity between Searles' earlier work and that of Csikszentmihalyi and Rochberg-Halton (1981) is indeed noteworthy. Each conceptualizes object relationships as symbols of the self representing and symbolizing the evolution of a personal identity, a sense of social belonging, and a connectedness with one's total world.

Csikszentmihalyi and Rochberg-Halton (1981) define and explain the role of object relationships in, for example, representing and symbolizing.

Power: The spear of the early hunter, the child's first tricycle, the 10-speed bike, and the motorcycle are some of the objects we can identify as representing power. One might also consider the sports car, the high-powered rifle, the race horse, "power dressing" of the 1990s, and the intellectual power of printed volumes, chessmen, or the Phi Beta Kappa key as representations of power.

Status is a dimension of power. Those objects associated with status are frequently the same as those symbolizing power. The most notable difference tends to be the cost and/or rarity of the object. This category might, therefore, include the expensive, sleek car, the large home with the five-car garage, the private jet, or the spacious, well-carpeted office. Carpeting as a status symbol was verified in an amusing and popular expression that circulated in Washington, D.C. some years ago. It was alleged that the power and status of a bureaucrat could be determined by the amount of static electricity generated by walking across the carpet. Objects that set the owner apart from the majority tend to signal status, such as the Super Bowl ring; the attaché case; collections of art, coins, and antique cars; and other special objects. Certain sports, such as tennis, cricket, and polo, represent status more than others do, such as baseball, basketball, or skating.

Objects are also identified as symbols of *social integration.* They serve to express dynamic processes within the self, among people, and between people. Those objects that people use and are engaged with are seen as representing the relationship of person to self, others, and the universe. Object relationships are, therefore, an integral part of the ongoing processes of defining self, differentiating self from other humans and one's one-human world, and connecting and integrating self with others and one's cosmic world. According to Csikszentmihalyi and Rochberg-Halton, the process of socialization is viewed as encompassing two central, inter-related, mutually reinforcing goals. These are stated as the differentiation of self and the integration of that self with others. At first glance, this may sound like a contradiction, a paradox. However, the knowing of self and one's uniqueness from others is a critical dimension for becoming socially integrated, for achieving a sense of inclusion, a sense of belonging. The similarity between Searles' earlier work and the more current publication of Csikszentmihalyi and Rochberg-Halton reinforces the descriptive role of object relationships in these processes.

This latter study adds knowledge and perceptions from the field of psychology, as well as extending a number of earlier constructs. Religion is described as a universal, social integrative symbol, particularly its associated objects and rituals. Those objects that are an integral part of shared group experiences, such as the Torah, Bible, Koran, crucifix, rosary beads, communion, songs, and prayers, all represent and symbolize belonging and differentiation. Through the ages, these and many other religious objects and rituals have represented and generated a sense of inclusion of being an integral member of one's social world. These shared experiences serve not only to represent the integration of self with others but also relatedness to one's cosmic world.

There are other objects and associated rituals in our daily lives that embody affiliation. Those secular objects symbolic of inclusion can be identified as, for example, team emblems on a sweater, cap, or T-shirt. Traditional awards and celebrations of graduation; rites of passage; special memberships; sports teams, contests, and the cheering crowds; national flags; and anthems are further examples that symbolize both differentiation and inclusion. Gifts and gift giving are viewed as representing a bond with others or the desire to bond. One very traditional example of the meaning of a gift is the engagement ring that signals belonging, the wedding ring as bonding. Other rituals that reflect some of the meanings of gifts and gift giving include, for instance, long-stemmed red roses as contrasted with a bouquet of spring flowers or the white lily plant. Christmas and Hanukkah gifts, the early religious sacrifices and gifts exchanged between the rulers or heads of countries.

Cultural differences are evident in the choice and use of objects at both a personal and social level. As we begin to study in subsequent chapters about activities associated with games, toys, sports, and crafts, for example, cultural differences will become more apparent. At this point, we can acknowledge that certain objects and their meanings are culturally specific, such as the crown jewels; the oval office; military bands, their dress codes, and cadence; wedding ceremonies and celebrations; holiday foods and rituals; and folk songs and dances.

According to Csikszentmihalyi and Rochberg-Halton (1981), the choice of objects not only reflects cultural differences but age differences as well. These differences can be understood by considering objects as comprising two categories: action objects and contemplative objects. Objects of childhood and youth are understandably action oriented. Examples in this category include the tricycle, bicycle, football, baseball, skis, skates, sports sneakers, etc. Contemplative objects are those that emphasize reflection and thought, such as books, fishing gear, musical discs, special object collections, photos, paintings, or crossword puzzles. Such objects are most frequently associated with late adulthood. During mid-life, object choice tends to combine both categories.

Comparing the special household objects of women with those of men in this study, it was found, not surprisingly, that men and women generally paid attention to different objects. On those occasions when the same object was valued, it was for different reasons. Men's preferences usually related to physical action and self needs. Women's choices reflected a broader parameter. Men, for example, identified their special objects as relating to their careers and leisure interests. The women's treasured objects centered on nurturance and interpersonal roles. These differences are corroborated by Kelly and Godby (1992) in their study of the etiology of leisure. Addressing the impact of the suburban lifestyle on leisure activities, they describe a "gender separation" in terms of choices. The activities of men most frequently center on sports and career-related object relationships. Women tend to be engaged in gardening and garden clubs, card playing, luncheons, and domestic-related activities.

The parameters of the Csikszentmihalyi and Rochberg-Halton study precluded exploration of object relationships in shaping and defining gender roles and identity. However, gender identity is a very significant part of self-identity, and engagement with objects is an influential dynamic in shaping and signifying gender. In Chapter 1, reference was made to activities that signal and/or symbolize gender and the related social roles expected in our western culture. Observations of the play activity of children and youth and the store displays and sales of toys and games reveal gender differences in object choice and behaviors. It seems fairly evident that the adult object preferences of men and women have their origins in the object relationships of childhood and youth. Action toys and objects most typical of boys have been found to relate to physical activity. The nurturing, caring objects are representative of the more frequent choice of girls. Physical maturation as well as culture are determinants in such gender differentiations. For example, hopscotch and jump rope, especially double dutch, have traditionally belonged to the activity repertoire of girls. Leg and lower body strength make it possible for the young girl to succeed and enjoy these activities. Boys, on the other hand, would be taunted by their peers if they chose such play (Henderson, Bialachki, Shaw, & Freysinger, 1996). Furthermore, boys would find such activity physically difficult. On the other hand, young boys' skill and enjoyment in baseball or football is congruent with their developing shoulder and arm strength.

The frequency of women's objects symbolizing caring and nurturing in contrast to the action-oriented object preferences of men are evident in girls' choice of dolls and toys related to home making, while the power toys and physical action games and toys are the most frequent choice of boys. These differences and their underlying sociocultural values have been discussed in a number of publications. Recently, Kaplan of *The Boston Globe* (1996) published an account of the annual New York Toy Fair. Boys' and girls' toys were explicitly displayed separately, and it was noted that the gender chasm in terms of expected toy preferences loomed wide as ever. The boys' section was filled with action toys, such as remote-controlled trucks, rocket firing products, Batman, Star Wars toys, Superman, and sleekly designed race cars. The toys for girls included a variety of dolls as well as Barbie and a complete shopping mall with beauty parlor, boutiques with glamour gowns, and a cash register that opened to accept the girls' gold cards.

These are pointed examples of how sociocultural values and their associated behavioral expectations are communicated and reinforced in object relationships. The apparent universal appeal and popularity of certain toys, automobiles and vans, objects of art, and the like are testimony to the symbolic messages of objects and the need of individuals to be seen as more like than different from their peers. Csikszentmihalyi and Rochberg-Halton (1981) concluded that individuals confirm their humanness through engagement with those objects that characterize civilized society. From this perspective, we can perhaps begin to better understand some aspects of the phenomenon of the vast popularity of certain objects, as well as the frequency with which the special self-related objects of individuals are similar to or like those of others.

Objects and our engagements with them quite obviously play a significant role in our socialization, in coming to define self as human, and in developing those perspectives, values, and behaviors that make differentiation and inclusion possible. *The Meaning of Objects Interview* (Form 4-1 on Page 44) was developed by Fidler as a supplement to *The Object History* to be used as a guide for engaging individuals in talking about their treasured objects. The purpose of such an interview at this stage of the learning process is to provide an experience that will facilitate application and confirmation of what has been learned about object relationships as well to add to perspectives and knowledge.

As we know, the efficacy of a learning experience can be measured by the extent to which the experience is shared with and compared to the experiences of others and is critiqued against and related to previous learning. Therefore, material derived from these interviews should be shared, compared, and contrasted with the object histories previously completed and should be related to the material presented in this chapter. This interview should be conducted with someone unknown to the learner.

Csikszentmihalyi and Rochberg-Halton (1981) have postulated that the significance of the meaning of objects can be explained as encompassing three modes of transactions: the aesthetic quality of the transaction, the channeling of psychic energy, and the outcome or goal of the transaction. The end product of the transaction is seen as confirming and defining self, self-other, and the cosmic self. We have been able to capture a glimpse of each of these as we have explored the theme of object meaning. As we move forward and broaden our study to include the total activity, these dimensions of engagement with the nonhuman environment will be more thoroughly addressed.

Form 4-1
THE MEANING OF OBJECTS INTERVIEW

Objects, or things, are very important in our everyday lives. They may represent a special interest, skill, event, belief, or value. They may serve as a reminder of an important person in our lives, or we may treasure certain objects because of their beauty, monetary or historical value, or because they make us feel good.

1. Among your important objects, which three are most special to you?
2. How did you come by each of these, and how long have you had each?
3. What is special about each?
4. How do your spouse or partner and children relate to these?
5. Are there possessions that have been important to you that you no longer have?
6. Does your spouse or partner have special objects different from yours?
7. How do these differ from yours?
8. What do you think are (were) your parents most treasured objects?
9. Taken together, what do all of your objects seem to mean to you?

REFERENCES

Csikszentmihalyi, M., & Rochberg-Halton, E. (1981). *The meaning of things: Domestic symbols and the self.* Cambridge, MA: Cambridge University Press.

Fine, S., & Fidler, G. S. (1971). *The object history.* Unpublished outline.

Henderson, K. A., Bialachki, M. D., Shaw, S. M., & Freysinger, V. J. (1996). *Both gains and gaps: Feminist perspectives on women's leisure.* State College, PA: Ventura Publishing Company.

Kaplan, F. (1996, February 17). Gender equality buried under toy fair aisles. *The Boston Globe.*

Kelly, R., & Godby, G. *The sociology of leisure.* State College, PA: Venture Publishing Company.

Searles, H. (1960). The nonhuman environment. New York: International Universities Press.

ADDITIONAL READING

Csikszentmihalyi, M. (1990). *Flow: The psychology of optimal experience.* New York: Harper Row.

Edwards, B. (1979). *Drawing on the right side of the brain.* Los Angeles: J. P. Tarcker.

Finan, C. R. (1982). *The ethnography of children's spontaneous play.* In: G. Spindler (Ed.). *Doing, The ethnography of schooling.* New York: Holt, Rinehart and Winston.

Gilligan, C. (1982). *In a different voice.* Cambridge, MA: Harvard University Press.

Deciphering the Message: The Activity Analysis

Gail S. Fidler

Developing an appreciative understanding of the many dimensions of meaning that are inherent in activities and coming to respect their role in shaping and reflecting human behavior is an intriguing and challenging endeavor. One important part of such pursuit is examining activity using a structured analysis. This involves critique of an activity's historical and current sociocultural inferences and meaning, its signs and symbols, and its physical and mental performance requirements. The end goal is to arrive at a discerning understanding of the character of the total activity. Understanding the ways in which a given activity or class of activities are similar to and different from other activities is a significant dimension of analysis. It is a comparative, evaluative procedure rather than a quantitative measure. For example, after the examination of an activity, one might conclude that its form and structure represents a higher degree of predictability and, thus, greater assurance against failure than activities A, B, or C, but less predictability than activities D, E, or F. This perspective is especially important in any undertaking aimed at matching a person or group to activity experiences.

One further concern is to ensure that an activity is analyzed and assessed in its own right. The purpose of an activity analysis is to arrive at an understanding of the activity's inherent qualities and characteristics, its meaning in and of itself, irrespective of a performer. Only after such an analysis has been made can one begin to discern the probable impact of an activity on an individual or group. Connecting or matching an activity to the needs, interests, and characteristics of a person or group requires a sophisticated understanding of both activity and person. Comprehending performance requires thorough knowledge of the characteristics of an activity, the characteristics of the person, and the dynamics of engagement.

In approaching activity analysis, it is important to keep in mind that an *activity* is defined as a sphere of interrelated actions that require the active engagement of an individual's mind and body in pursuit of the goal or end product of such action. A *task*, on the other hand, is a segment of an activity and comprises the lowest performance level of the whole. For example, combing and brushing one's hair or buttoning one's blouse are tasks within the activity of personal grooming. Parking a car is a task within the activity of driving, and "making a shot" is a critical task of the activity of basketball. An activity is viewed as encompassing form and structure, properties, action processes, outcome, and realistic and symbolic meanings and inferences within each of the five elements and in the total activity.

There are a number of different perspectives that influence how activities are studied and assessed. In therapeutic recreation, activity analysis is taught and used as a prerequisite for program planning. Activity analysis is viewed as a procedure for examining the inherent characteristics of activities to select those most appropriate to program objectives. Analysis includes assessment of the cognitive, physical, interpersonal, social, affective, and administrative factors. The outlines and ratings scales for such analyses are impressively thorough and are a valuable resource for the study of activity analysis (Peterson & Gunn, 1984; Avedon, 1974).

In contrast, adaptive physical education usually examines activities by means of task analysis. This procedure involves the examination and ordering of the tasks that comprise an activity, rather than the activity as a whole. The purpose of this process is to facilitate and guide the teaching and training for skill acquisition (Wuerch & Voeltz, 1982). The approach of education to the study and examination of activities is likewise one of task analysis. This procedure is used primarily in special education, job training, and vocational programs. The process involves defining and grading the sequential steps that comprise the given tasks of an activity in order to provide a protocol for teaching those skills that are necessary for mastering a given course of study (Wolery, 1996).

Activity analysis and task analysis reflect different perspectives and intentions. Activity analysis is a process that assesses the elements or characteristics of an activity for the purpose of identifying and defining the dimensions of its performance requirements and its social and cultural significance and meanings. It is a process of looking at parts as these relate to defining the whole. Task analysis, on the other hand, is concerned with identifying the sequential steps of a given task within an activity, breaking down these tasks into steps or building blocks that can be taught and that will result in the acquisition of skills and related performance. This procedure addresses the actuality of tasks and, as such, does not customarily include consideration of sociocultural, subjective, or symbolic dimensions.

Since its early beginnings, occupational therapy has included activity analysis in its education and practice. Initially, the procedure was similar to a task analysis with a focus on the physical movement aspects of activities for their remedial value. Creighton (1993) reported that crafts were evaluated in terms of what joint motion and muscle strengthening they provided and required. These perspectives were broadened earlier by Haas (1922) in the published activity analysis, which addressed the social and emotional needs aspects. Some 20 years later, Fidler published an activity analysis outline with an emphasis on psychological factors (Fidler, 1948). This analysis has been updated several times (Fidler & Fidler, 1954 and 1965) with the most recent revision appearing in this chapter.

Since the 1970s, the profession has witnessed a plethora of published approaches to activity analysis. The perspectives reflected in these have been to assess and analyze an activity on the basis of its therapeutic and restorative uses. These analyses are, therefore, closely related to the authors' frame of reference regarding therapeutic intervention within a special area (Allen, 1985; Cubie, 1985; Cynkin & Robinson, 1990; Llorens, 1978; Mosey, 1986). More recently, the American Occupational Therapy Association's *Uniform Terminology* has been used as a basis for analysis (Cottrell, 1996). A positive spin-off from this approach seems to be a broadening of scope toward a more generic frame of reference. This broadened or more holistic perspective is evident in more recent publications (Breines, 1995; Lamport, Coffey, & Hersch, 1996; Watson, 1997). However, there are inherent pitfalls in using the *Uniform Terminology* as a basis for activity analysis. It is indeed difficult to translate aspects of performance into elements of an activity without compromising or distorting the activity. Activities in and of themselves do not contain elements or characteristics of self-expression, coping, self-concept, and the like. These reside within the person, not within the activity. This differentiation is addressed by Nelson in his artful description of occupation and the distinction among the activity itself, the performance, and the dynamic of performance (Nelson, 1988). When activity analysis is primarily a procedure for determining the applicability of an activity or its tasks for particular therapeutic or rehabilitative purpose, there is high risk of overlooking important aspects of an activity's "character." When task analysis is the principle approach to the assessment of activities, the risk of losing sight of the multidimensional dynamic of the total activity is heightened.

A quite different point of view for critiquing the characteristics of activities is suggested in the research of Moore and Anderson (1968). In their seminal study, these scientists concluded that the socialization of the human being could be explained as developing, in part, out of experiences with certain types of games and activities. Certain activity characteristics were seen as corresponding to characteristic attitudes and perspectives that a person needed to develop in order to function adequately in his or her world. The folk model paradigm created by these scholars offers an intriguing dimension to the study of certain aspects of activities. Four classes or categories of games/activities were identified by Moore and Anderson. These encompassed puzzles, games of chance, strategy, and aesthetic entities. These were classifications used by them to structure learning environments, and they were not intended to be a format for the analysis of activities. However, the relevance is obvious, and, some years ago, I took the liberty of using their perspectives as a basis for looking at activities in the following way.

PUZZLES

Included in the puzzle group are those games and activities that contain most of the principle elements and characteristics of a puzzle. We can conjecture that such activities and games would, thus, contain a high degree of form and structure, predictable outcomes, clear procedures and sequencing, parts that are clearly related to a whole, and limited action alternatives.

Was the crayoning activity in the laboratory primarily a puzzle activity? From this viewpoint, how is it like or different from the collage? What other activities fit the puzzle category? Knitting? Working the computer? Working crosswords? Bookkeeping? In what ways?

One significant factor of this classification is that the performer can control and predict the outcome.

Games and Activities of Chance

The principal factors in games of chance are that these are the opposite of puzzles. Elements of form and structure, such as rules and procedures, are few and do not ensure predictable outcomes. Cause and effect relationships and results are capricious and "iffy" at best. The performer is the recipient of consequences beyond his or her control. Games of blackjack, poker, and roulette are a few examples.

What other activities contain significant elements of chance, keeping in mind that the salient characteristic of chance activity is the unpredictability of outcome? In what ways and to what degree do the finger painting and collage activities of the laboratory experience fit this category? How might the following be compared in terms of elements of chance and puzzle: fishing, playing Scrabble, running a race, hunting, bowling, and abstract oil painting?

Games of Strategy

These are characterized by the inclusion of a significant other. These are activities in which all actions and outcomes are influenced and determined by the interplay of two or more people. The action of each participant is planned and carried out on the basis of the plan and action of the other. These are games and activities characterized by needing to know or anticipate as much about the other as one knows about one's own plan of action. Included in this classification are, for example, team sports, chess, checkers, bridge, and tennis.

How do these compare with, for example, golf, Parcheesi, folk dancing, bike racing, and hide and seek?

Aesthetic Entities

This category is less well-defined and, therefore, is more difficult to apply to the process of analyzing activities. However, this element references those activities that require making evaluative judgments, those that call into play the role of the umpire, judge, or referee. Evaluative judgments are an essential part of activities, such as performing a music, art, or drama critique, museum curator, or sports refereeing. Additionally, we might consider a number of careers and jobs as requiring a significant degree of evaluative judgments.

Which ones could be included here? What about collecting special objects? Judging one's end product of an activity?

Most activities contain a mix of puzzle, chance, strategy, and judgment. However, each comprises more of one characteristic than any other. Assessing where an activity seems to fit on such a scale can certainly enrich one's perspective and discernment.

The following activity analysis outline includes those revisions that have been made over time to more readily ensure that the analysis would focus on a critique of each of the five elements of an activity and, thus, facilitate coming to understand that activities do indeed have meaning in and of themselves. The approach to this analysis is explained in part by the following descriptions.

FORM AND STRUCTURE

The elements of *form and structure* significantly determine the quality and extent of an activity's predictability of processes and outcome. The amount of insurance against failure can be measured by the extent of an activity's structure, the clarity and thoroughness of its rules and procedures, the degree to which these guard against chance and, thus, ensure a predictable outcome or product. The similarity to puzzle activity is evident. In making a comparative evaluation, one might, for example, contrast and compare the crayoning activity in the laboratory experience (see Chapter 3) with operating a computer or perhaps compare the form and structure of knitting a sweater with a game of chess and a game of bingo. Each of these activities has clear and explicit procedures and rules that must be followed.

Which aspects make a difference and reduce or increase the predictability of action processes and outcome, actually or inferred?

PROPERTIES

The properties of an activity—the objects, materials, equipment, space, setting, and people—define the "character" of an activity to a significant extent. This segment of an analysis is concerned with the assessment of the nature of each property and its impact on defining and characterizing the activity. For example, a setting, such as a library, gym, baseball field, classroom, or television room, communicates certain functional purposes, cultural meanings, and inferences that then elicit subjective associations. An analysis assesses these and considers the ways in which such meanings and inferences help to define the character of the activity. For instance, materials that are pliable and, thus, are readily responsive to actions of the performer, such as the paint or ball of clay, knitting wool, or bread dough, communicate expectations and meaning quite different from hard, resistive objects or materials such as a block of wood, sheet of metal, volleyball, treadmill, or pulleys.

The question is what inherent meanings are generated and reinforced by the properties and in what ways? In reference to Chapter 4 and the discussion of objects and their meanings, what objects are part of the activity and what can be said about their significance and meaning?

Equipment and objects that are manipulated by hand project sociocultural and personal messages quite different from those that are power driven.

What are the differences among the wooden toy truck that must be pushed by hand, the wind-up truck, or the one with the remote control? In terms of the interpersonal dimension, does the activity require the engagement of more than one person? What social roles and relationships are necessary? How do games of strategy apply here? How does the

"person" aspect of the activity compare, for example, with a team sport, the game of triv-
ia, blackjack, or the quilting bee?

Recently, at a craft fair, a craftsman was making and displaying braided rugs. He had designed and was using a small device that braided the strands of wool, eliminating the slower procedure of braiding by hand.

How is this activity changed? Is it now a different activity? In what ways?

ACTION PROCESSES

The focus in this section of the analysis involves identifying and evaluating the varied actions and the psycho-motor behaviors that are essential for reaching the end goal of an activity. This examination addresses those actions that call into play sensorimotor function, cognition, psychological structure, and interpersonal processes.

The principle question is which behaviors of each of these domains are necessary and at what level of skill? Furthermore, how does each compare with the requirement of other activities?

If, for example, one were to evaluate the circle ball toss activity in the laboratory experience (see Chapter 3), a conclusion might be that higher levels of balance, muscle strength, and gross motor coordination were required than in walking, planting a flowerbed, or bathing, but less than is necessary for jumping rope, in-line skating, or riding a bike. One can explore, for instance, how the action elements of puzzles, chance, and strategy contrast among a game of bingo, checkers, scrabble, or bridge.

Assessing the cognitive requirements of an activity could involve a comparison with those necessary for a game of chess, creating a collage as in the laboratory experience, budgeting one's income, and surfing the Internet. Psychologically, base functions might possibly be evaluated by contrasting the extent of external control (rules, regulations, patterns, umpire, etc.) among dressing for a day at work, styling one's hair, jury duty, and waiting tables. The element of competition can be understood by perhaps comparing this aspect of the activity with playing Monopoly, tennis, bowling, deep sea fishing, and dressing for a costume party. Finally, the nature of interpersonal strategies necessary for engagement in a given activity might be compared with playing basketball, playing poker, managing a department, ballet dancing, and conducting an orchestra.

OUTCOME

The *outcome* or end product of all activities, like other elements, has actual as well as symbolic meanings. The material presented in Chapter 4 that explored the many dimensions of meaning in objects is particularly relevant to the study of the significance of outcome. In most instances, the significance of a given outcome varies according to both culture and time. Even a casual glance at local and national newspapers and television will confirm the value placed on winning or losing outcomes. This is especially evident in organized, competitive sports. Even during international Olympic games, the winning points and scores of nations frequently take precedence over individual achievement, thus reinforcing the inclusion-exclusion dynamic.

The influence of time and the sociocultural changes it brings is evident in how objects and end products are and have been viewed. A decade or two ago, tennis outcomes had far less widespread significance and popularity than is true today. Over the years, soccer outcomes have continued to be seen as less important in the United States than in Europe. Needlecraft products were highly valued prior to the mid-20th century but have significantly declined in value since then. For example, embroidered pillow cases, crocheted antimacassars, smocked aprons, and dresses are objects of the past.

In contrast, what are some of the highly valued outcomes and end products of today? What are the comparative social, cultural, and subjective meanings and inferences of, for instance, the end product of a vegetable garden, a flower garden, figure skating, a string ensemble, a barbecue, and a wine-tasting event? In what ways do outcomes and end products signify belonging and/or differentiation? What are some examples?

REALISTIC AND SYMBOLIC MEANING

Several of the previous chapters have set the stage for examining the questions raised in this section of the outline. This process calls upon an understanding that has developed from exploring the dimensions of metaphor and symbol throughout history and in one's everyday life. The questions posed in this part of the analysis should trigger associations with material presented in earlier chapters, with other literature, and with one's own daily living experiences and folklore.

We have seen that each element of an activity as well as the total activity has realistic literal meaning and significance. These elements also represent, at a symbolic level, sociocultural values and beliefs as well as personal associations and inferences. Therefore, to truly understand the full nature of an activity, it is necessary to explore and critique all of these dimensions.

The primary goal of this section is to identify and examine the symbolic representations, the subliminal messages inherent in the objects and properties, and the action processes and outcome of an activity, and then to compare and contrast these with other activities. This procedure generally involves identifying and describing the literal, functional meaning of the elements of an activity, then to ask what inferred, symbolic statement is contained in each. For example, a pattern with clear explicit rules for its use has as its purpose ensuring that the outcome, the end product, will be what was intended. At a symbolic level, the pattern and rules and procedures may symbolize and infer predictability, very limited risk, control of outcome, and protection against failure.

In dealing with this section of the analysis, it is important to remember that there are no absolutes. The search for meaning is just that, a search for an exploration. As Fine reminds us in Chapter 2, "while there are predictable themes that define and challenge, there is no prescription for determining meaningfulness" (p. 12). Several examples should help to clarify this process of examining and exploring meaning—the inherent subliminal messages, if you will.

One of the questions in the outline asks how the aggressive and/or destructive actions of the activity are controlled actually and symbolically. Depending on the activity, one might cite examples of actual control as existing in the rules of the game that prohibit body contact, or the inclusion of a referee, or the pattern that must be followed, the instructions for using the hammer to drive the nails, or the saw to shape the wood. Symbolically speaking, these realities give messages of external control, of forces outside of self that prevent loss of control or the aggressive action being contained.

How agreement on the nature of reality is evident at a realistic and symbolic level can be illustrated by using the example of the activity of playing in a marching band. The first step is to look at all of the major elements of the activity's rules and procedures, objects, actions, and outcome or end product. Thus, one might itemize such realities as the musical score, managing the instrument in tune and in accordance with the music sheet, keeping time and rhythm, cadence, marching formations, responding to the band leader, identical uniforms, etc. Then, the second step is to ask how and in what ways do these realities enable the performer to sense, to feel, to experience, in a figurative sense, being in tune, being out of tune, in step, or out of step with others, as well as to associate the experience with belonging, sharing others' reality, and validating self as real and more connected than not. In further exploring the symbolic dimensions of activities, one might compare and contrast making a dress from a pattern, playing in a basketball tournament, driving a taxi in Los Angeles, and playing pinochle.

What are the different dimensions of the properties, actions, procedures, and outcomes of each? How might the nature of external control be described in each, and what makes the difference? What elements are similar? How are their interpersonal dimensions alike and different? What can be said about outcomes, about predictability, and about the sociocultural meaning and significance of the total activity? How have these meanings changed in the past decade or two?

SUMMARY

This final section provides a general descriptive summary of the principle characteristics of the activity as compared with a sampling of other activities. This summary description, while not limited by those features in the outline, should at least address each of these.

Analyzing activities and coming to a perspective about their characteristics and nature is a qualitative, descriptive process. Any evaluation and assessment is a comparative analysis. There are extremely few, if any, absolutes in such a process and a great many "more or less" and "as compared to" conclusions.

ACTIVITY ANALYSIS OUTLINE

The following is designed to guide the learner through the process of coming to know, understand, and respect an activity in its own right, as having meaning in and of itself. An activity analysis is concerned only with the study of the activity itself, its actual and symbolic characteristics, its sociocultural significance, and how these define the "character" of the activity.

An activity is viewed as comprising five interrelated elements: form and structure, properties, action process, outcome, and actual and symbolic meanings at social, cultural, and personal levels. An activity analysis is the process of assessing and evaluating these elements, comparing them with the same elements in other activities to arrive at a comparative analysis of the total activity and its parts.

1. **Form and structure:** The nature and extent of rules, procedures, time elements, and sequences required in the activity.
   a. How extensive and explicit are the rules and procedures that must be followed?

b. Are these patterns to be followed or reproduced? To what extent?

c. Are there a few or multiple procedures to follow?

d. To what extent, if any, can these external controls be altered or disregarded without significantly changing the activity and goal? What freedom to create is possible?

e. Do patterns, rules, and procedures define and/or mandate a sequential process? Provide sequenced steps for achieving the end goal?

f. What are the time elements? How important are these to sequence and the end goal?

g. Other characteristics relative to describing form and structure?

h. How does the nature of form and structure compare with other activities?

2. **Properties:** The objects, materials, equipment, people, space, and setting required.

a. What objects, materials, equipment are required?

b. What are the characteristics of each: size, pliability, responsiveness, rigidity, resistiveness, texture, color, etc.?

c. What sociocultural meanings are represented in the objects, the materials, and the equipment?

d. To what extent does the activity require involvement of more than one person? How many and in what roles?

e. What is the nature of the space and setting that is required?

f. What symbolic messages are reflected in the required space and in the setting?

g. How do these properties compare with those of other activities?

3. **Action processes:** The kind and nature of the actions (the psychomotor behaviors) that are necessary for carrying out the activity.

a. What sensorimotor behaviors and at what level are required?
   - Balance and equilibrium
   - Visual perception
   - Tactile discrimination
   - Spatial awareness
   - Visual-motor integration
   - Language and hearing
   - Fine motor coordination
   - Gross motor coordination
   - Muscle strength and endurance
   - Physical force
   - Other

   How do these physical integrity and skills requirements compare with other activities?

b. What cognitive behaviors and at what level are required?
   - Time management
   - Retention and recall
   - Sequencing
   - Computation
   - Cause and effect discrimination
   - Attention span
   - Reasoning and problem solving
   - Judgment

- Ideation and creativity
- Other

How do these cognitive requirements compare with those in other activities?

c. What psychologically based behaviors and at what level are required?

- Coping with ambiguity
- Coping with external controls
- Managing risk
- Postponing gratification
- Coping with competition
- Assertion, aggression
- Other

How do these behaviors compare with the requirements of other activities?

d. What interpersonal behaviors and at what level are required?

- Awareness of the other
- Shared planning
- Cooperation and shared performance
- Role delineation and clarification
- Other

How do these behaviors compare with the requirements of other activities?

4. **Outcome:** The end products, the outcome expectation of the activity.

a. What end product is inherent in the activity?

b. What meaning and value does society place on this outcome?

c. What sociocultural meanings are represented in the end product or goal of this activity?

5. **Actual and symbolic meaning:** The reality-based and symbolic components of the total activity and each of its parts #1 through 4, form and structure, properties, action, and outcome? What comparisons can be made with other activities?

a. What value does society place on this activity?

b. What are some of the symbolic meanings of this activity in today's society? In times past? How are these similar to other activities?

c. What is and what has been the gender identification of this activity, of its properties, and action processes?

d. What is the comparative age relevance and association of this activity and each of its parts at a realistic and symbolic level with other activities?

e. What is the nature and extent of opportunity for self-expression?

f. To what extent is performance dependent upon internal ideation and creative thinking? In what ways?

g. What is the nature and opportunity for invention or alteration?

h. To what extent is the process representational or reproductive rather than creative?

i. What is the nature and extent of external limits and controls? Realistically and symbolically?

j. What opportunities exist for the performer to be in control? Realistically and symbolically?

k. To what extent and in what ways do form, properties, and action processes provide control, set limits, or provide assistance? Realistically and symbolically?

l. What is the frequency of repetition, of changing processes?

m. To what extent and in what ways do action processes involve motor behaviors that are primarily aggressive, assertive, or passive? Directly and symbolically?

n. In what ways are the aggressive and/or destructive actions controlled or managed, realistically and symbolically, in form and structure, in properties, in action processes, and/or in end product?

o. To what extent and in what way do structure, properties, and action processes provide opportunity for agreement on the nature of reality? Realistically and symbolically?

p. What opportunities, at a realistic and symbolic level, are there for the performer to identify personal contributions and efforts?

q. What is the nature and extent of opportunity to test the reality of one's perception?

r. What is the nature and extent of opportunity to be dependent on a person or structure? Realistically and symbolically?

s. To what extent and in what ways are objects, structure, and processes symbolic of childhood dependency?

t. In what ways, realistically and symbolically, is there opportunity for independent performance or autonomy?

u. What is the potential for and nature of competition?

6. **Summary:** A descriptive summary of the following principal characteristics of the activity and how each compares with similar characteristics in a sampling of other activities.

a. Social/cultural meaning and value

b. Gender orientation

c. Age relevance and association

d. Contemplative—action focused

e. Inclusion—differentiation

f. Autonomy—external controls

g. Predictability—chanciness

h. Creativity—structure

i. Cognitive level

j. Physical skills

k. Solo performance

l. Group/team performance

REFERENCES

Allen, C. K. (1985). *Occupational therapy for psychiatric disease.* Boston: Little, Brown, and Co.

Avedon, E. M. (1974). *Therapeutic recreation service: An applied behavioral approach.* Englewood Cliffs, NJ: Prentice Hall.

Breines, E. B. (1995). *Occupational therapy activities from clay to computer.* Philadelphia, Pa: FA Davis.

Cottrell, R. P. F. (1996). *Purposeful activity: Foundation and future of occupational therapy.* Bethesda, MD: American Occupational Therapy Association.

Creighton, C. (1992). The origin and evolution of activity analysis. *Am J Occup Ther, 46,* 45-48.

Cubie, S. H. (1985). Occupational analysis. In G. Kielhofner (Ed.). *A model of human occupation: Theory and application.* Baltimore: William and Wilkins.

Cynkin, S., & Robinson, A. M. (1990). *Occupational therapy and activities health: Toward health through activities.* Boston: Little, Brown, and Co.

Fidler, G. S. (1948). Psychological evaluation of occupational therapy activities. *Am J Occup Ther, 2,* 284-287.

Fidler, G. S., & Fidler, J. W. (1954). *Introduction to psychiatric occupational therapy.* New York: MacMillan.

Fidler, G. S., & Fidler, J. W. (1965). *Occupational therapy: A communication process in psychiatry.* New York: MacMillan.

Haas, L. G. (1922). *Occupational therapy for the mentally and nervously ill.* Milwaukee, WI: Bruce Publishing.

Lamport, N. K., Coffey, M. S., & Hersch, G. I. (1996). *Activity analysis and application: Building blocks of treatment* (3rd ed.). Thorofare, NJ: SLACK, Incorporated.

Llorens, L. A. (1978). Activity analysis for cognitive—perceptual—motor function. *Am J Occup Ther, 27,* 453-456.

Moore, O. K., & Anderson, A. R. (1968). *Some principles for the design of clarifying educational environments.* Pittsburgh: University of Pittsburgh, Learning Research and Development Center.

Mosey, A. C. (1986). *Psychosocial components of occupational therapy.* New York: Rover.

Nelson, D. L. (1988). Occupation: Form and performance. *Am J Occup Ther, 42,* 633-641.

Peterson, C. A., & Gunn, S. L. (1984). *Therapeutic recreation program design: Principles and procedures.* Englewood Cliffs, NJ: Prentice Hall.

Watson, D. (1997). *Task analysis.* Bethesda, MD: American Occupational Therapy Association.

Wolery, M. (1996). Using assessment information to plan intervention programs. In: M. McLean, D. B. Bailey, Jr., & M. Wolery (Eds.). *Assessing infants and pre-schoolers with special needs.* Paramus, NJ: Prentice Hall.

Wuerch, B. B., & Voeltz, L. M. (1982). *Longitudinal leisure skills for severely handicapped learners.* Baltimore: Paul H. Brooks.

ADDITIONAL READING

Kielhofner, G. (1997). *Conceptual foundations of occupational therapy.* Philadelphia: F. A. Davis.

Codes of Meaning: Play, Games, and Sports

Beth P. Velde

The differences between the occupations of play, games, and sport lie in both their substance and meaning. For the purposes of this chapter, we will accept the premise of Guttman (1988) that play is the overriding term that encompasses these three activities. Two categories of play are spontaneous play and organized play or games. Within games, there are noncompetitive games and competitive games or contests (Table 6-1). Contests may consist of intellectual contests or physical contests that include physical games and sports. A characteristic common to all of these is that they are done for their own sake. One becomes involved in them or stays involved in them for intrinsic reasons. While there are those who initiate or continue to do them for extrinsic reasons, such as health, fitness, academic credit, or pay; the intrinsic pleasures of the activity for the person are what seem to distinguish it as play as opposed to work.

PLAY

Huizinga (1995) characterizes play as voluntary, encompassing the freedom to become engaged, remain engaged, and to terminate one's engagement at one's own discretion. Secondly, play involves suspension from reality. The play requires the focus of the player within the activity to the extent that reality is suspended and the concentration of the player is focused upon the moment. As Huizinga (1995) sug-

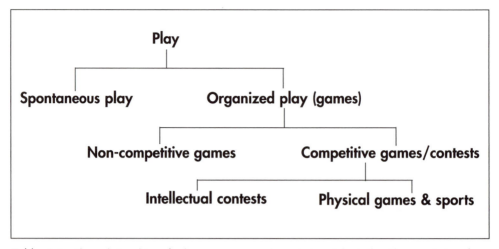

Table 6-1. The relationship of play, games, and contests. Adapted with permission from Guttman, A. (1988). *A whole new ball game* (p. 2). Chapel Hill, NC: University of North Carolina Press.

gests, "play presents itself to us ... as an intermezzo, an interlude in our daily lives" (p. 6). However, this does not mean that play is not serious. What occurs during the play engagement is both meaningful and purposeful to the player. The seriousness of play is obvious to anyone who has become so involved that he or she loses track of time.

A third characteristic that is frequently included as a distinguishing characteristic of play is that, in its separateness from ordinary life, it assumes its own space and time. Play occurs within a set or predetermined physical space. This can be the playground, the card table, or the football field. Even in spontaneous play, in which there is less structure accorded, the players define a portion of physical space as the areas that will be used. Think of the child playing dress up with mommy's high heels and make-up or with daddy's coat and tie. He or she sets aside a portion of the physical space of home as the place where this play will occur. This ordering of experience represents the opportunity to control one's world, to change it, to be an equal.

Similarly, play has a beginning and an ending. Time has a different dimension in the play experience in that the focus of time is on the immediate experience. Worrying about tasks not yet accomplished or words uttered yesterday have no place in the play encounter. The players are engaged in the here and now. When hunger interferes or the expectations of others intrude, the play experience is ended, and the player is returned to other tasks of daily life.

This use of space and time creates a structure in the play experience. While the ordinary world may lack order for the player, play places the determination of order upon the player. Play, by its nature, allows the individual to manipulate the experience to maintain novelty. When the skills and abilities of the player match the requirements of the play activity, he or she can change the physical space or the time, creating an element of chance. This chanciness continues the tension between the player's skills and abilities and the requirements of the play activity. Ellis (1973) suggests that this opportunity for manipulation of the experience provides the player with avoidance of boredom.

Many theorists believe that intrinsic motivation is a key characteristic of play. Some authors suggest that for the player to be intrinsically motivated, the activity must have elements of freedom, and the player must be in control of his or her participation. Sutton-Smith (1986) proposes that this characteristic ties into the work ethic prevalent in Western society. Work is obligated, and the motivation for participation is external. Elements of freedom are constricted and the worker has relatively little control over his or her participation. When play is defined as the opposite of work, key characteristics of play revolve around issues of freedom and control. This bears further thought because it implies that playing completely resides within the control of the individual. This does not account for the role of the environment, both human and nonhuman. For example, in regard to the nonhuman environment, is it possible that the environment and the objects in it "press" the individual into play?

Think of the child on a playground. Which comes first, the child's desire to play at the playground or the playground's "invitation" to play? What about the play involved in rituals and ceremonies? Or the play that occurs during portions of social time, such as recess at school? Moore (1990) attempts to further understand the role of the environment in the development of play in children. She suggests that an accompanying concept to Huizinga's *homo ludens* is her concept of terra ludens. This is her attempt to explain the phenomenon of the reciprocal reactions between player and environment and the responsibility of the player to the environment.

Sutton-Smith also suggests that the characteristic of intrinsic motivation as part of play is not as instrumental as a defining concept in developing countries or those with lower socioeconomic classes as it is among the play researchers. Finally, in today's world, children are socialized into an educationally based system early in life. At two, they are attending preschool programs, and even younger children are involved in daycares that foster play as a means of learning. "Do we idealize children's play as freedom, as a compensation for our own guilt in giving them so little leeway or alternatives to compensate ourselves for having so little?" (Sutton-Smith, 1986, p. 43).

Play is dissimilar to other types of occupations in its use of irrationality. Occupations of self-care, jobs, careers, and education are viewed as using rationale means to achieve an end and, therefore, are frequently labeled by society as serious. In contrast, play sets up artificial barriers between the goal and achievement of the goal. The rules of play increase the chanciness and risk inherent in play. Therefore, it is frequently viewed by society as being symbolically less serious. Play is detached from the continuity of daily life on both a figurative and symbolic basis. Play activities are not real life, and they mostly stay without real consequences for serious existence (Scheuerl, 1986, p. 20). In a similar manner, play allows the player to connect his or her fantasies and his or her imagination to reality. The player is able to actualize impulses and test the possibilities and limitations of reality and vice versa (Herzka, 1986) without serious consequences.

Play has changed in the United States. Before World War II, sandlot play was accepted and occurred frequently. After World War II, play became more organized, and sports opportunities for children increased. This fit well with an industrialized society that was compartmentalized and where adult lives were structured around work. It symbolized the structure of the work world and reinforced the belief that effort and hard work pay off in success. Yet, many fear the organization of play sends deeper messages to children—that musing, "playing around," and creating are not valued in our society.

Esposito (1974) asserted that games and sports, in general, may be perceived as "contrived situations, the purpose of which is to heighten and bring into focus the interplay between possibility and actuality" (p. 141). For example, one does not need to run a marathon or play football to exist. But the contriving of the experience allows the player the opportunity to test his or her skills and knowledge and determine what he or she is capable of through the actual doing of an occupation.

Feminist authors have argued that men have completed much of the research and writing about play. As such, play theory has been biased by a predominantly male perspective. This has been particularly evident in the lack of research on collaborative play, verbal play, and the fleeting moments of play evident in the play experience. Authors such as Babock (1978); DeKoven (1978); Fluegelman (1976); Henderson, Bialeschki, Shaw, and Freysinger (1996); and Schwartzman (1978) indicate that play must be understood within its context. Social interactions, relationship to the environment, personal history, role expectations, gender identification, race/ethnicity, and social class all relate both to how play is understood and how play development occurs within individuals. As such, the focus upon individualistic nature of the player described in much of the play literature must be challenged.

The role of spontaneous play in the formalized educational system has been relegated to the early childhood programs. Our culture does not view this type of play as something that should occur in school beyond these early years. While the play of childhood is viewed as amusing, it is not seen as part of the learning process (Lakin, 1996). In contrast, games appear to be used more frequently in elementary schools as a way to learn and practice academic concepts and physical skills. This is, in part, due to the increased amount of structure inherent in the games and their adaptability to academic goals. However, there is some evidence that, among minority members of our society, even games are not considered a legitimate part of the formal educational process. African-Americans, Hispanics, and Asian immigrants are striving to share the opportunities of the majority. For them, education is linked with and symbolic of success and the opportunity to achieve at least middle-class status. Play at school symbolizes a lack of seriousness toward the goals of some of these individuals for their children (Lakin, 1996).

The use of games in schools for the fostering of academic concepts further separates this type of play from the spontaneous play described above. Play in this case focuses on cognitive development and ignores the uniqueness of play as a holistic experience. When experienced by the player, play should be felt as a total experience. The mind does not direct the body any more than emotions drive the thinking process. The experience occurs as one to the player. When play and games are used without this understanding, the experience becomes less play-like and loses many of its features described earlier. It further splits the player into parts and focuses on the part valued by, in our case, the industrialized, achievement-oriented society where intellectual abilities are a key to success.

Play Environments

Recent theorists in geography have suggested that environments and landscapes play a major role in the construction of identity (Cosgrove, 1985; Cresswell, 1996). This concept bears reflection in regard to play. For example, the reaction of society when women enter an environment formerly controlled by men (such as the female reporter in the football team locker room) conveys messages regarding femininity and masculinity. The reading of the meaning behind society's questioning of this behavior has a lot to do with the acceptance and reproduction of an ideology of female roles. Likewise, the designation by parents of a "play room," by teachers of a place where recess activities take place, and by planners of a park area carries messages that play occurs apart from everyday life. Within these play environments, the landscape is frequently constructed in a way that rules and expectations of society are adhered to. Hence, places become associated with concepts, such as masculine and feminine—the football field versus the dance studio.

Spontaneous Play

Many different types of play experiences occur within spontaneous play. These include sensorimotor play, such as sand and water play, dramatic play, toy play, and interaction with technology. However, there appear to be times when at least some of these experiences may not meet the characteristics of play described above. When the young child interacting with the action figures from a popular television show mimics the actions seen on television, critical elements of the play experience are missing. Using the toys as props in a repetition of the television program, the child brings little of his or her own experience into the play activity (Levin, 1996). However, if the same child using the same objects creates his or her own scenario, the experience would more closely resemble play.

Play provides the opportunity for exploration and the discovery of the potential and capabilities of the player. It allows the player to exhibit power and control. For example, building stilts not only enables the player to discover if his or her carpentry abilities match the demands of the occupation and if his or her understanding of physics is complete enough to manage the stilts in order to walk, the stilts themselves enable the player to tower over his or her peers, to appear more powerful than his or her playmates.

Toys lend themselves to diverse types of play. Blocks and Legos demand construction-based activities. Rattles, beads, and puzzles require manipulation. Dolls, doll beds, play furniture, and appliances offer representational play. Dramatic play is encouraged through clothing, settings, such as a storefront, and the provision of puppets.

Toys have always carried messages about reality that represented the dominant class. In a discussion of antique toys, Ketchum (1981) reviews a variety of toys and reveals to the readers some of the symbolism associated with them. He states,

> *They strongly reflect accepted contemporary mores—that little boys should be brave, honest, and hardworking, that little girls should be kind, dutiful, and attentive to their elders. And they reflect, too, the prejudices that existed at the time they were produced. Games like "Alabama Coon" and mechanical banks denominated "Paddy and His Pig" or "Chinese Must go" reveal such feelings all too clearly.* (p. 7)

Meier and Murrell (1996) caution observers of spontaneous play among children to carefully interpret the children's play with objects. As children develop, they acquire the ability to see objects as "standing for" something else, as symbolizing something else. In acquiring this ability, their play becomes more imaginative and allows for a more sophisticated use of objects, concepts, rules, and roles. However, too often, the observer assumes that the child's symbolic interpretation of an object is the same as the observer, without taking into account the cultural context of the player. The observer must acknowledge his or her own assumptions and biases regarding both the material object and the symbolic representation. The reader should refer to the discussion in Chapter 4 on the language of objects and to the discussion of the activity laboratory in Chapter 3 for further examples. The players' assignment of sign and symbol to play objects is dependent on their own personal experiences. Hence, if a child has not experienced using a ticket to travel on a train or airplane, it will be difficult for him or her to see a slip of paper as a sign for a ticket or a symbol of freedom. Similarly, Meier and Murrell caution the reader to determine whether Barbie serves for the child as a symbol of sex identification or as "a prop for the enactments" of children as "future selves as women and lifelong friends" (p. 103).

One of the most frequently discussed objects of spontaneous play is the doll, especially Barbie. This may stem from the possibility that doll play among young girls fosters and reinforces stereotypical sex roles and an unrealistic body image. Barbie's portrayal of the ideal feminine body as having disproportionately large breasts and thin waist and hips may further exploit, through symbolism, what the ideal American female should look like. By the same token, young boys continue to play with action figures, trucks, and sport objects. Again, both the objects and the play symbolically reinforce the role of men in North American society. Would changing the objects of play change the messages? Perhaps. But are parents of today ready to have boys engaging in traditionally female play activities? As Pollitt (1995) explains, "Could it be that even sports-resistant moms see athletics as part of manliness? That if their sons wanted to spend the weekend writing up their diaries, or reading, or baking, they'd find it disturbing? Too antisocial? Too lonely? Too gay?" (p. 22).

Recent research has suggested that toys that are associated with some aspect of adult social structure continue to show the greatest gender difference in children's preferences for toys. Freeman, Sims, Kutsch, and Marcon (1995) suggest that changes in toy preferences occurred in those toys used mostly for personal enjoyment. Girls are as likely as boys to enjoy riding bicycles and engaging in some type of sports. Boys are as likely as girls to participate in arts and crafts, games, and music. However, play objects, such as military toys and dolls, which orient children toward representational roles of social structure, still show gender differences. The real question arises in the power of these toys symbolically. How much influence does the toy itself have on stereotypical behaviors and roles? Or is it society itself that imbues in children at an early age the preference for these toys because of the role models and media messages the child perceives?

Every plaything symbolizes the totality of real things, yet the plaything yields to the player in a way that the real world does not. Play endows everyday things with a sense of magic. Children exhibit attachment to objects of play (and self-care). They take the doll, blanket, soother, or stuffed animal everywhere they go. It is possible that this object has become a symbol of their manifested, objective self. Leaving the object behind would be like leaving a part of themselves behind.

Spontaneous play includes the use of playground equipment. Remember the thrill of the slide—being in control at the top and letting yourself go as you began your descent? Or remember the heady feeling of vertigo as you spun around and around on the merry-go-round? It also involves the use of the environment to create hidden spaces—houses, nests, secret places that become safe havens for the players. Here, the player represents his or her world and orders it according to his or her rules. While the play experience may reflect real life and carry the substance of everyday experience, the player knows at the same time that it is make-believe. The card table is draped with a cloth and becomes a house. The player brings in objects that stand for the furnishings. He or she plays out the roles of mother, father, sister, brother, friend, and enemy in a safer place. While it may symbolize the outside world, it provides a rich opportunity for the development of an inner self.

Perhaps no one describes the joy and value of spontaneous play better than Erickson (1977):

> *To truly play, you must learn to use the ground as a springboard, and how to land resiliently and safely. It means to test the leeway allowed by given limits; to outdo and yet not escape gravity. Thus, whenever playfulness prevails, there is always a surprising element, surpassing mere repetition or habituation, and at its least suggesting some virgin chance conquered, some divine leeway shared.* (p. 17)

To better understand the role of play in your life, consider the questions on Page 66 and respond as completely as possible. Compile a narrative of your play history to this point in your life. Reflect upon your history in relationship to the points raised in this chapter. How has your play been influenced by your gender, environment, personal history, culture, and significant others? What does this say about the characteristics of play relative to yourself?

GAMES

One of the characteristics that distinguishes a game from spontaneous play is the establishment of a recognized and agreed upon goal among a large group of people. This goal frequently involves beating other players (to win) or mastering the environment (to score at or under par on the golf course). Suits (1995a) suggests that for either goal to retain a lusory attitude, the goal must be accomplished within the rules of the games, in a sportsmanlike manner. The text of the game consists of the rules of the game and the physical setting in which it occurs. The rules of the game prescribe the means by which the goal can be accomplished. This includes the objects to be used, the rules of fair play, the means by which the goal can be accomplished, the penalties for breaking any of the rules, and the role of the player. In spontaneous play, many of the same characteristics may be present, but these characteristics are determined at the time of the play by the players involved. Hence, when young children play dress up and Amy is assigned to be mommy, this role of player is set at the time of the dramatic play. The objects prescribed in playing mommy, the dress, and the roles the players assume are assigned by the players. (However, many would suggest that these are "prescribed" by society through the role models and the media.) When players join together in a game of soccer, cards, or Monopoly, the constitutive rules of the game are set and understood prior to the game encounter. Games also consist of a context, the social setting for and meaning of the game to both the players and society.

Games provide a means for the players to further self-interpretation. Through their engagement in the game, they both judge and perceive themselves—their skills, abilities, and view of themselves—relative to others involved in the game.

NONCOMPETITIVE GAMES

In Chapter 5, Fidler introduced the work of Moore and Anderson, who suggest that games may take on four modes: puzzles, chance, strategy, and aesthetics. Within each of these categories, the players take on different roles. Games of chance are not competitive, at least relative to another player. Sutton-Smith (1986) suggests that games of chance "vie

PLAY/ACTIVITY HISTORY
by Gail S. Fidler

I. Identify and describe those games or activities in which you engaged most frequently during these four periods of your life: preschool years (ages 0-5), grade school years (ages 5-9), pre-adolescent years (ages 9-13), and adolescent years (ages 13-17). These should be the activities that you remember when reflecting on each period of time and may include experiences in which you participated on a regular basis and/or were events to which you looked forward.

II. For each period of time, choose one play activity and explain a.) who taught you the activity; b.) what you recall as the most enjoyable aspect of the activity; c.) with whom you most frequently shared this activity (such as mother, father, sibling, friend, self, other); and d.) the extent to which this activity was part of your family's culture (played by them or their parents) and/or part of your peer culture, and/or unfamiliar to parents/family/peers.

III. Of the four upon which you just elaborated, which do you recall as the most enjoyable, the least enjoyable? Why?

IV. For each of these four, relate the activity to your stage of learning and development by describing the specific practice and learning that the activity provided for you in such areas as:
   - sensory-perceptual skills
   - motor skills
   - self-identity, self-concept
   - cognitive skills
   - dyadic skills
   - group skills
   - testing of reality
   - meeting your needs

V. For each of the four, describe the elements of puzzle, games of chance, strategy, and aesthetics that exist in the activity. For each of the four activities, which element seemed the most dominant?

VI. Describe each of the four activities you chose in terms of the following aspects:
   - its competitive elements/cooperative elements
   - the relative amounts of gross motor and fine motor demands
   - the relative time spent in participant and observer roles
   - the relative amount of structure versus creative or unstructured elements present

For each activity, which of these did you find most enjoyable, least enjoyable?

with physical contests as amongst one of the most primary meanings of the concept of play" (p. 51). Here, games of chance are seen as a symbolic means of learning to deal with the irrevocable conflicts of social reality. This is especially apparent in the work of Geertz (1978), who suggests that the game of cock fighting and its accompanying gambling among the people of Bali is a way for members of that society to understand what would happen if all of society was allowed to assume the same behavior and direction. Sutton-Smith (1986) interpreted Geertz's view: "In participating, one can literally lose one's gambling shirt, but most participants can become knowledgeable about deeper truths of their own society" (p. 52).

Games of chance and lotteries were generally perceived negatively and were denied widespread social or legal approval until recently, largely because they contravened the accepted norms requiring concerted efforts and dedication for the attainment of rewards. When those rewards switched from the individual player to potential productive aspects for groups in society (such as reduction of tax monies and use of lottery dollars to support seniors programs), social acceptance was gained.

CONTESTS

Games of strategy reflect a higher level of complexity in society. These games appear to involve power struggles and deception. Moore and Anderson claim that games of strategy teach about the importance of a significant other—the need to know as much about the other as you know about yourself. Many suggest that games of strategy serve as a metaphor for social reality. However, there appears to be one large difference. By nature of their definition, games involve constitutive rules that constrain the struggles encountered. Rules regarding fair play attempt to discourage any type of social breakdown from occurring. This appears in contrast to real life.

INTELLECTUAL CONTESTS

Contests that predominantly use cognitive skills include board games, card games, word games, and video games, among others. Video games have been designed to mimic aspects of the real world. Early games emulated sports such as tennis (Pong), auto racing (Pole Position), or military combat (Missile Command). More recently, games more accurately simulate real life occupations such as golf, fishing, football, and fantasy exploration, such as the exploration of alien planets (Super Metroid), castles (Kings Quest), and cartoon adventures (Super Mario).

The content of the games often carry messages not obvious to the player. For example, one of the original video games was Pac-man. In an effort to appeal to a feminine audience, its producers developed Ms. Pac-man. Here, the original character was transformed from a small, male, yellow character to one with female characteristics including lipstick, hair bows, and long eyelashes. More recent video games designed to appeal to the feminine market incorporate female leads who are presented as rugged and capable, using both strength and intellectual skills. However, these games lack the action-oriented, violent, and aggressive characters usually seen in games that are designed for the male market. According to Delp (1997), "This type of game (the thinking game) has generally been considered more appealing to the female audience than fast-paced, violent games, supposedly preferred by male players" (p. 28).

Many of the action-oriented games have male leads usually seen as heroes. Women are typically portrayed as individuals who can only survive with the help of the lead male. Sometimes, women are included as a backdrop to the theme of the video game, though frequently in roles that are less powerful than the male lead. These games carry powerful messages to their players about the attributes of men and women.

Some of the more recent and more controversial fighting games, such as Mortal Kombat and Street Fighter, include women characters who take an active role in fighting against other characters in a tournament-style contest. Players are free to choose the characters they wish to use from a group of characters. However, the big, brawny, white men still predominate. The pool of characters also includes a few other racial identities, such as Asians, African Americans, and Native Americans. This may be a sign that game manufacturers are increasingly aware of a minority market for their games. It may also symbolize an increasingly androcentric nature to society's perception of violence, power, and physical strength. However, some would caution that this is really a masculinization of female characteristics in an attempt to create both a higher level of sales and a masculine norm for society.

What is interesting among the video games available to the retail market is the lack of characters who are older or disabled. This, too, carries messages to the player about who possesses strength and power in our society.

Card, table, and board games also depend on cognitive skills for the player to be successful. While chance may play a part in some board games, such as rolling the dice in Chutes and Ladders, Monopoly relies on both chance through rolling the dice and strategy regarding purchasing properties and using game cards. The content of board games frequently symbolizes the predominant values of the day. Initially, book learning (*Journey through Europe* or the *Play of Geography*) and religion and morality (*The Game of Pope or Pagan* or the *Siege of the Stronghold of Satan* by the Christian Army) were stressed. In the late 1800s, material success became valued, and the game of business and speculation were introduced. These were followed by the ultimate game of material success—Monopoly.

Chess has long been regarded as the ultimate game of strategy. Destruction appears to be the soul of the game. Its theme deals with the fates of kings and queens. Yet, like Christianity, the lowly pawn has the opportunity to become the stuff kings are made of (Avedon & Sutton-Smith, 1971). The role of the queen in chess changed over time and appears to symbolize the changes that real women of power underwent in relationship to history. Chess provides warfare that is organized, controlled, circumscribed, regulated, and socially approved. It further has symbolic representation of the great players of social history—the king, queen, priest, general, sage, and philosopher. It is a game of both skill and reason that emphasizes thinking over more primitive physical acts of aggression and may symbolize the values accorded to cognitive skills in today's society. Chess highlights the role of the significant other in games of strategy and the relationship of one player to another.

In a similar manner, the table game of cards represented the society of the ruling class when they were first introduced. Spades represented nobility; hearts represented clergy; diamonds represented merchants; and clubs represented peasants. Players of bridge and poker will recognize how these games use those signs to symbolize the predominant social structure of the day (and some would say of today).

PHYSICAL GAMES AND SPORT

Many of the games of childhood involve physical skills but are not the true test of the body that sport is considered to be. Jacks is one example. Jacks involves rhymes, bouncing the ball, and picking up as many jacks as one can. It includes messages of friendship. In contrast, among the Brazilian Indian tribe Yanomamo, there is a punching game in which a male player attempts to see how tough he is and how much pain he can endure from punches thrown by fellow tribesmen. To the Yanomamo, this is a ritualized game that forms an integral part of the system that determines adult male social status. Punching games exist among American men as well, though they tend to be more playful in nature. However, this type of game still serves to identify power and dominance among the players.

A seemingly universal content for games are the hiding and seeking games. These begin with peek-a-boo and continue on to hide-and-go-seek and capture-the-flag. All such games may create in the players a sense of being wanted. The young child hiding behind his hands and the older child hiding under the bed is sought by another. This occurs within a safety zone established by the rules of the game. In peek-a-boo, the child is seen yet unseen by the other player. Peek-a-boo for the infant is symbolic of the other always returning.

In hide-and-go-seek, the player ventures further into the world. The hiders share a similar plight, being sought by the person who is "it." Strategy and deception are necessary to stay successfully hidden. Yet, each hidden player anticipates the stalker and relishes being found and joining the social group again. This may represent a desire that all humans share—to be seen, to be missed, and to be separate from and together with other people.

Other games appear to be relics of ancient rituals. Hopscotch is believed to be an extension of the ancient labyrinths and later was adopted to show the soul's journey from earth to heaven. In one lay-out of the game, the base square from which one starts is labeled earth and the circle toward which one is striving is labeled heaven. Party games such as drop the handkerchief, spin the bottle, or post office are considered extensions of ancient fertility rites.

Juggling is a game that involves keeping several objects in motion in the air simultaneously by tossing and catching. The objects may be balls, bean bags, handkerchiefs, or Indian clubs. The activity requires dexterity and manipulation skills, along with coordination. Juggling was considered a form of harmless entertainment and dates back to the times of royalty when juggling provided entertainment for kings and queens. Juggling is a game of dynamic balance in which controlled equilibrium must be accomplished to keep the objects from falling to the floor. Juggling today serves as a euphemism for life itself. People talk about juggling a number of activities but remaining in control. Bookkeepers "juggle the books" to steal money without being caught.

Juggling also represents overcoming hardships in human existence, "... a world where things fall down and apart," but the talented individual (the juggler) achieves a balance and maintains control of life. Juggling is associated with Doctor Faustus, one of the renowned jugglers and con artists of history. He is portrayed as someone who puts himself in harmony with gravity to overcome the entropic workings of the world. Likewise, juggling is symbolic of men's and women's existence, where the world may be seen as operating on a delicate balance out of their control, where there are rings kept spinning by the master juggler balancing on the firmament of time (Chandler, 1998, p. 3).

Physical games and sports share many attributes. They allow the player to push himself or herself physically, psychologically, emotionally, or cognitively in a way that is not possible in everyday life. Perhaps, for some, they simulate man's earlier life when competition against nature predominated. They may allow adventure in a world that is nonadventurous, routine, sedentary, and noncompetitive. This may occur through playing the game or vicariously through watching the game or remembering past experiences. Games may incorporate power or finesse in the style of play and position of the player. Many require a physical sensitivity—the ability to shoot a free throw, complete a set shot in volleyball, putt in golf, throw the stone accurately in hopscotch, or hit the marbles with the shooter. Physical games also involve both physical and psychological risk. How a player approaches these may symbolize his or her approach to risk in real life. Does he or she play conservatively to minimize strategic risks? Does he or she avoid pressure situations to decrease emotional risks? Physical games are also a sensuous experience. The smell of a baseball glove, the sound of a ball hitting the metal bat, the visual poetry of a well-turned double play, and the exaggerated sound of the heartbeat as the hidden player anticipates being found in hide-and-seek all create essential parts of the game experience. The kinesthetics of coordinating body parts shares similarities to dance. Chapter 10, *Voices of the Arts*, provides a more detailed discussion of this concept.

Sports differ from physical games in that they are predominantly games of physical skills that are widely understood within a particular society. They involve testing the body and a sense of communality. There is a group of followers who are typically called fans. Lastly, there is some stability regarding the constitutive rules and understanding of these rules by both players and fans. Suits (1995a) suggests that this stability fosters both attendant roles (such as coach) and institutions (such as the National Collegiate Athletic Association or Professional Golfers' Association). These foster the training and development of athletic skills, research, development, and coaching.

Sport and its accompanying training and skill development has been linked with health. This link with a "serious" goal may be viewed as a way for a society still caught up in the "work" ethic to view sports as worthwhile. Fitness and the desire to be in shape may also serve as a euphemism for the desire to be physically attractive. Sport and fitness activities allow participants to enjoy, to feel pleasure without guilt.

Recent writing has described an objectification and denunciation of the body in sport. The body is viewed as a machine, and programs have been dedicated to and obsessed with reification, efficiency, and productivity of the body in the pursuit of excellence. This may be tied particularly to male sport in which athletic fields become the places where the development of physical presence, stoic courage in the endurance of pain, and superior judgment create the man. Male sports frequently celebrate the differences between men and women, particularly in the form of competition that favors power, aggression, and domination. Think of football, rugby, hockey? Even sports that originally penalized power and aggression (such as baseball and basketball) find more of their players fined and suspended for fighting, pushing, and being physically dominant during the event. This supports concerns about society's increasing preoccupation with violence. When women engage in many of these traditionally male-dominated sports, they are frequently labeled as confrontational and aggressive, traits associated with masculinity.

Baseball has become a symbol to those living in the United States as a representation of the American culture. It has been viewed as an expression of hard work, moral integrity, and self-discipline often associated with the American dream. This can be further exemplified when examining some of America's heroes. For example, Mickey Mantle, despite his problems with alcoholism, was seen as one such hero. His blond hair and blue eyes helped to serve as symbols of the "All-American Boy." Despite his inconsistencies at the bat, he symbolized America's uncomplicated youth. Football players are frequently viewed in a similar manner. As participants in a sport in which power and strength dominate, this activity represents the veracity of the saying "survival of the fittest." Sabo (1994) describes his perspective as a football player: "When we ball players, clad in fiberglass armor, made our triumphant entrance into the stadium, they would cheer and feel their values were still intact. America was still beautiful. Young men still struggled against one another. Competition reigned supreme" (p. 14).

Athletic fields themselves may be symbolic of the American culture. Here, people impose their will for order upon nature. Greenskeepers are in charge of the natural grass and "cut the grass every day." This despite the fact that "the higher you keep the grass, the healthier it is" (Zwaska, 1998). If the grass begins to turn brown or wears away so the dirt shows, greenskeepers paint the area with green paint. When natural turf is seen as unmanageable, artificial turf is installed. Order is further prescribed by the contrast of the white lines against the clay of the infield or the green of the field. Looking at an athletic field that has been well kept symbolizes control and dominance over the environment and signifies social structure.

Golf has long been viewed as the domain of men. The golf course was both a place to compete and a place to do business. Golf clubs frequently limited women's memberships, women's playing privileges, and women's access to club facilities. The same treatment was accorded to minorities. When women and minorities were allowed to play, they were frequently subjected to signs and symbols of their unwelcomeness. The golf ball that barely missed the woman poised on the green to putt sent a clear signal: Women don't belong on the golf course. This behavior may have its roots in the era when women stayed home. Men, the argument went, needed exclusive rights to lunch hour and weekend tee times because they were the only hours they didn't work. In addition, men use golf for the serious business of wooing clients and discussing work with clients. In contrast, women were accepted on the tennis court, where, clad (until recently) in white dresses, they observed the decorum and manners expected of the female gender.

Golf has also been viewed as a sport of integrity and manners. This is enforced even among spectators during tournaments through the use of course marshals and fore caddies. Like the players, spectators are expected to display appropriate behavior, with "contained enthusiasm" the preferred behavior.

In the past, women were prohibited from participating in or were marginalized from many sports. Sports were viewed by society as a test of the body. Due to perceived anatomical and physiological differences, women were more accepted in sports requiring accuracy, skill, and grace. Culturally, this seemed to protect women from being harmed or disfigured. This resulted in a truncated view of women's sports, in which women were allowed to participate in the same sports as men except where undue dangers existed. However, participation was frequently limited by additional constitutive rules that further protected them, such as in girls' basketball. Another strategy was to use a handicapping approach in order to "scale" women to men. Women themselves questioned the value of participation in some sports, fearing loss of femininity and social appeal.

Aggressiveness and the devaluation of women is further symbolized in the language associated with male sport. This includes the verbal sparring that occurs among the players, such as "you throw like a girl" or "faggot." Locker rooms still include sex talk and graphic descriptions of sexual exploits. Lastly, sports metaphors permeate the language of sexual conquest with talk of "scoring" or "getting to second base."

More recently, signs and symbols of women's acceptance into the sport arena are appearing. It wasn't long ago that the *Sports Illustrated* swimsuit edition was the only place women were seen in the sports media. Recently, the changing view of women's body image has been symbolized in *Women's Sport and Fitness*, a publication not unlike *Sports Illustrated*. Women are increasingly seen engaging in physical contests throughout the popular media, the Women's National Basketball Association has achieved national broadcast rights.

Elite players of sport also use their status to flaunt predominant cultural values. Dennis Rodman may be one such example. His nickname is "The Worm," an interesting metaphor. Worms are usually viewed as symbols of death, connected with lowness, vileness, and contempt. Sometimes, the worm is understood as a symbol for the penis. Rodman's behavior also may symbolize a lack of adherence to conformity and societal expectations. Being late for practice, striking officials and photographers, and foul language on the court all are examples of going against the rules and regulations imposed by the sport of basketball. His public appearance, which includes tattoos, multicolored hair, and cross dressing seems to be an attempt to further draw attention to himself. Yet, he continues to be acknowledged as one of the best players in basketball, and his physical training is well known among fans. (Many would say his antics are really an act, a way to draw attention from the fans.) He serves as the perfect foil to his fellow teammate, Michael Jordan. Jordan follows the rules, acts courteously toward others, and dresses in a way accepted by society. His nicknames include signs of royalty, such as "His Airness." Together on the same team, they serve to play the symbolic roles of hero and villain.

Ritual and ceremony also play a large part in the messages that sports carry. The singing of the national anthem and presentation of the flag remind us that sport has a political context. Ceremonies also serve as a method for preserving and symbolizing affiliation, especially in international events. The playing of the anthem at the Olympics, World Cup, and World Series symbolizes the affiliation of the winning individual or team with a particular country.

Objects, including uniforms, protective equipment, and sports equipment, are frequently viewed as symbols of allegiance and belonging. Some sports equipment allows the player to do more than the player could do with his or her bare hands, feet, head, or legs. The player must accept his or her body and unite it with items beyond it, getting the feel of the equipment through constant use. Every player tries to get to the point in which the equipment becomes part of him or her, to where he or she hardly notices it. Through this act, the body is extended beyond the point at which it normally can function. When this occurs, an identification of the player with his or her equipment exists. He or she feels masterful and in control. This allows him or her to effectively carry out the role in situation after situation, where he or she is adjusted to whatever else is there and is, thereby, enabled to perform with and through them excellently. In turn, others see this player as successful, competent, and at home in the world, whether this be the world of common sense or the more restricted worlds of business or sport.

Spectator Sports

An alternative to actual participation in sport is sport viewing. While observers of this phenomenon still struggle to understand the hold it has taken on American society, it nonetheless has created a multibillion dollar industry. Spectator sports incorporate live viewing, television, computer access, and radio. The aspect of spectating affects both the performer and the viewer. According to Cozens and Stumpf (1953), "Beginning with the accomplishments of early childhood and extending up through the highest achievements of civilizations, one of the strongest incentives to perfection, both individual and social, is the desire to be praised and honored for one's excellence" (p. 284). Coupled with this is the cultural aspect arising from the American society's valuing of achievement. As such, recognition and eminence is "coveted, not disparaged," and such "eminence must be earned and not created by the social structure itself" (p. 285). In an attempt to identify with the sports heroes, fans don T-shirts and other objects of identity.

Some scholars suggest that athleticism has qualities of aesthetics. The actions of sport carry elements of poise, balance, contrast, variation, rhythm, and harmony. The viewer of athletic events is a skilled observer. As a fan, he or she understands the skill and techniques used to execute the sport. Frequently, his or her knowledge may have begun as a player and, as such, is based (at least to some extent) on first-hand experience. Many spectators become experts, aware of specialty skills, training, statistics, and players' history, using these in judging performance.

Sport spectating also bears many of the characteristics of play discussed earlier. Becoming immersed in watching allows the viewer to escape the reality of everyday life. If viewing in person, he or she is able to alter his or her environment and to experience all the sensory stimulation associated with sitting in the stands. Think of the smells, noises, sights, tastes, and physical sensations of attending a baseball game, tennis match, or football game. While the observer does not get the same type of emotional release the player may experience, he or she often reports a change in feelings. Vocal participation, active cheering, and verbal (and sometimes physical) sparring with opponent fans may all be part of the activity characteristics of fan participation. For many who are no longer physically or psychologically able to play the sport, this may be the only way to participate. It also provides a sense of community through a shared experience. This is reinforced through characteristics of the vicarious experience itself, such as fan clubs, websites, sports broadcasters, and promotional materials that serve to identify the fans to each other.

Anyone who has ever attended a Denver Broncos football games knows to look for the Bronco barrel man. Fans dress in team colors, wear face make-up that accentuates team symbols, and chant team mottos. All serve as symbols of belonging. Sport figures are frequently seen as heroes, and my team becomes the "good guys," while the opponents serve as the "bad guys." Individual links with greatness are symbolized in the autograph, picture, or foul ball caught during a major league baseball game.

Television and radio as a means for spectators to observe a sport also carry messages. The limited coverage (at least until recently) of women's sports and sports involving people with disabilities carries a strong message regarding importance and value. This may be especially true when women and individuals with disabilities are seen as weak or imperfect. A second message often conveyed by the media is the importance of the individual. While television and radio may cover team sports, they frequently highlight the performance of the "heroes" and may well do features of these individuals during breaks in play. Television and radio cover sports using announcers who serve as narrators of the event. These announcers serve to educate the less-informed viewer, personalize the event, and interpret the event. As such, the narrative serves to mold the symbolic message being portrayed. Frequently, the message is "anyone can compete and that stereotypically attractive women continue to watch physically powerful men play the game" (Cantelon & Gruneau, 1988, p. 191).

ASSUMPTIONS ABOUT PLAY

Too often, in the discussion of play, whether it be spontaneous play, games, or contests, individuals assume that humans play in order to learn. How many times have you heard someone suggest that "play is the work of childhood"? Yet, in play based on the characteristics discussed in this chapter, cognitive learning and physical skill development are not the pay-off the player is seeking. The engagement in the play experience comes from the process of the play. In spontaneous play, novelty and new experiences often occur serendipitously. Repetition of these experiences may lead to mastery of certain skills, but the goal of the player is not focused on learning. In a similar manner, the player of games and contests participates for the sake of engagement. During this engagement, it may become clear that, in order to create and successfully deal with elements of chanciness and novelty, he or she needs to alter elements of the engagement. This may occur through refining physical and intellectual skills, altering the constitutive rules, changing the nonhuman environment and the objects in it, or changing the humans who share the game experience with him or her. Again, while learning may occur, it is secondary to the engagement in the play experience. Refinement of skills and behaviors always relates to the process for accomplishing the goal specified for that particular game.

When play becomes externally controlled, is it still play? When the physical education teacher structures a class to "learn new skills," when the therapist has the child with a disability interact with others in a therapeutic play experience to assist in rehabilitation, when the parent structures a child's free time with endless periods of instruction, is play occurring? In these instances, the game becomes secondary. When this occurs, the opportunity for freedom and intrinsic motivation becomes compromised. Why is it that this occurs? Perhaps because play became a symbol of the antithesis of work. In a society dominated by the Protestant Work Ethic, play for its own sake was devalued.

PERSONAL REPERTOIRE: SECONDARY OCCUPATION

by Gail S. Fidler

The term secondary occupation refers to those activities that occupy an individual's discretionary time, those devoted to the pursuit of personal enjoyment and satisfaction. This category comprises those activities related to self-obligation—the sports, games, hobbies, and related activities of personal interest. This chapter has introduced you to the concepts of sports and games. The following chapters will include other activities that are frequently perceived as secondary occupations. Think about the following questions. Identify your responses in point form below each question. Write a narrative describing your repertoire of all your secondary occupations to this point in your life.

1. Briefly describe your current hobbies and activity interests.

2. How would you categorize each in relation to the following qualities?

Active _____ Passive

Participant_____ Observer

Competitive _____ Cooperative

Gross Motor Skills _____ Fine Motor Skills

Free Expression _____ Structure

High Level of Cognitive _____ Low Level of Cognitive

Skill Required   Skill Required

High Degree of Social _____ Low Degree of Social

or Cultural Relevance   or Cultural Relevance

High Interpersonal/ _____ Low Interpersonal/

Social Level   Social Level

3. What motivates you to be involved in these hobbies/activities?

4. Which is/are your favorite(s)? What aspects make each special?

5. How frequently are you involved in each?

6. What factors limit your involvement? What factors enhance your involvement?

7. How are these similar/different from your childhood activities? How are these similar/different from your primary occupation?

8. On the basis of the above, how would you characterize your activity profile?

References

Avedon, E., & Sutton-Smith, B. (1971). *The study of games*. New York: John Wiley & Sons.

Babock, B. (Ed.). (1978). *The revisable world*. Ithaca, NY: Cornell University Press.

Cantelon, H., & Gruneau, R. S. (1988). The production of sport for television. In: J. J. Harvey & H. Cantelon (Eds.). *Not just a game: Essays in Canadian sport sociology* (pp. 177-194), Ottawa, Canada: University of Ottawa Press.

Chandler, A. (1998, August 13). *Essay on the symbolism of juggling*. http://www.juggling.org/js/8714/symbol.html.

Cosgrove, D. (1985). *Social formation and symbolic landscape*. Totawa, NJ: Barnes and Noble Books.

Cozens, F. W., & Stumpf, F. S. (1953). *Sports in American life*. Chicago: The University of Chicago Press.

Cresswell, T. (1996). *In place/out of place: Geography, ideology, and transgression*. Minneapolis, MN: University of Minnesota Press.

DeKoven, B. (1978). *The well played game*. New York: Anchor Books.

Delp, C. A. (1997). *Boy toys: The construction of gendered and ritualized identities in video games*. Unpublished doctoral dissertation. East Carolina University, Greenville, NC.

Ellis, M. (1973). *Why people play*. Englewood Cliffs, NJ: Prentice Hall.

Erickson, E. (1977). *Toys and reason*. New York: W. W. Norton.

Esposito, J. L. (1974). Play and possibility. *Philosophy Today, 18,* 137-146.

Fluegelman, A. (1976). *The new games book*. New York: Dolphin.

Freeman, G., Sims, T., Kutsch, K., & Marcon, R. A. (1995). *Linking gender related toy preferences to social structures*. Savannah, GA: Paper presented at the annual meeting of the Southeastern Psychological Association, March 1995. (ERIC Document Reproduction Service No. ED 383 480).

Geertz, C. (1978). *The interpretation of cultures*. New York: Basic Books.

Guttman, A. (1988). *A whole new ball game*. Chapel Hill, NC: University of North Carolina Press.

Henderson, K. A., Bialeschki, M. D., Shaw, S. M., & Freysinger, V. J. (1996). *Both gains and gaps: Feminist perspectives on women's leisure*. State College, PA: Venture Publishing.

Herzka, H. S. (1986). On the anthropology of play: Play as a way of dialogical development. In: R. van der Kooij & J. Hellendoorn (Eds.). *Play, play therapy, play research* (pp. 23-34). Amsterdam, Netherlands: Swets North America Inc. International Symposium, September, 1985. (ERIC Document Reproduction Service No. ED 287 553).

Huizinga, J. (1995). The nature of play. In W. J. Morgan & K. V. Meier (Eds.), *Philosophical Inquiry in Sport* (pp. 5-7), Champaign, IL: Human Kinetics.

Ketchum, W. C. (1981). *Toys and games*. Washington, DC: Cooper-Hewitt Museum.

Lakin, M. B. (1996). The meaning of play: Perspectives from Pacific Oaks College. In: Playing for keeps: Supporting children's play. Topics in early childhood education, 2. (ERIC Document Reproduction Service No. ED 405 101).

Levin, D. (1996). Endangered play, endangered development: A constructivist view of the role of play in development and learning. In: Playing for Keeps: Supporting Children's Play. *Topics in Early Childhood Education, 2.* (ERIC Document Reproduction Service No. ED 405 104).

Meier, T., & Murrell, P. C. (1996). They can't even play right! Cultural myopia in the analysis of play: Cultural perspectives on human development. In: Playing for Keeps: Supporting Children's Play. *Topics in Early Childhood Education, 2.* (ERIC Document Reproduction Service No. ED 405 106).

Moore, R. C. (1990). *Childhood's domain: Play and place in child development*. Berkeley, CA: MIG Communications.

Pollitt, K. (1995, October 8). Why boys don't play with dolls. *The New York Times Magazine*.

Sabo, D. (1994). The best years of my life. In: M. A. Messner & D. F. Sabo (Eds.). *Sex, violence and power in sports* (pp. 11-15). Freedom, CA: The Crossing Press.

Scheuerl, H. (1986). Some phenomenological aspects of play. In: R. van der Kooij & J. Hellendoorn. *Play, play therapy, play research* (pp. 17-22). Amsterdam, Netherlands: Swets North America Inc. International Symposium, September, 1985. (ERIC Document Reproduction Service No. ED 287 530).

Schwartzman, H. (1978). *Transformation: the anthropology of children's play*. New York: Plenum.

Suits, B. (1995). The elements of sport. In: W. J. Morgan & K. V. Meier (Eds.). *Philosophical inquiry in sport* (pp. 8-15). Champaign, IL: Human Kinetics.

Sutton-Smith, B. (1986). The metaphor of games in social science research. In: R. van der Kooij & J. Hellendoorn (Eds.). *Play, play therapy, play research* (pp. 35-66). Amsterdam, Netherlands: Swets North America Inc. International Symposium, September, 1985. (ERIC Document Reproduction Services No. ED 287 553).

Zwaska, P. (1998, April 5). Why the grass is so green. *The Washington Post*, p. C3.

ADDITIONAL READING

D'Agostino, F. (1988). The ethos of games. In: W. J. Morgan & K. V. Meier (Eds.). *Philosophical inquiry in sport* (pp. 42-49). Champaign, IL: Human Kinetics.

Kerr, J. H. (1986). Play, the reversal theory perspective. In: R. van der Kooij & J. Hellendoorn (Eds.). *Play, play therapy, play research* (pp. 67-76), Amsterdam, Netherlands: Swets North America Inc. International Symposium, September, 1985. (ERIC Document Reproduction Service No. ED 287 553).

Kew, F. (1997). *Sport: Social problems and issues*. Oxford, England: Jordan Hill.

Kretchmar, R. S. (1994). *Practical philosophy of sport*. Champaign, IL: Human Kinetics.

Kretchmar, R. S. (1995). From test to contest: An analysis of two kinds of counterpoint in sport. In: W. J. Morgan & K. V. Meier (Eds.). *Philosophical inquiry in sport* (pp. 36-41). Champaign, IL: Human Kinetics.

MacNeill, M. (1988). Active women, media representations, and ideology. In: J. J. Harvey & H. Cantelon (Eds.), *Not just a game: Essays in Canadian sport sociology* (pp. 195-212). Ottawa, Canada: University of Ottawa Press.

Meier, K. (1988). Triad trickery: playing with sport and games. In: W. J. Morgan & K. V. Meier (Eds.). *Philosophical inquiry in sport* (pp. 23-35). Champaign, IL: Human Kinetics.

Saberge, S., & Sankoff, D. (1988). Physical activities, body *habitus*, and lifestyles. In: J. J. Harvey & H. Cantelon (Eds.). *Not just a game: Essays in Canadian sport sociology* (pp. 267-286). Ottawa, Canada: University of Ottawa Press.

Sansone, D. (1988). *Greek athletics and the genesis of sport*. Los Angeles: University of California Press.

Suits, B. (1995). Tricky triad: games, play, and sport. In: W. J. Morgan & K. V. Meier (Eds.). *Philosophical inquiry in sport* (pp. 16-22). Champaign, IL: Human Kinetics.

CHAPTER 7

Codes of Meaning: Nature's Challenge

Beth P. Velde

Nature has long been viewed as *Mother Nature* and referred to in the feminine tense. This has implicated a focus on its organic cosmology. More recently, nature has been seen as a resource or a commodity—something to be managed. This perhaps fits better with a mechanized and paternalistic view of the world. Occupations that occur in the natural environment reflect both of these perspectives.

When nature is viewed as a birthing or nurturing mother, she is seen as an entity that provides for the needs of all people. Activities that occur in the natural environment are done in a respectful manner. In contrast, a second image of nature as female casts her as wild and uncontrollable, one that "could render violence, storms, droughts, and general chaos" (Merchant, 1998, p. 278). It is this second perspective of nature as female, coupled with the mechanization of the modern world, that led to the belief that nature was a commodity, a resource to be mastered and controlled.

This chapter will focus on occupations that are best done outdoors and for which a major focus of the experience depends upon the natural environment. This focus may result from a need to overcome the environment or relate to the challenge of the environment, or it may result from a desire to be in tune with it. Such activities may involve alternative modes of travel, such as hiking, canoeing or kayaking, skiing, or swimming. Lastly, the geography may vary from mountains, to lakes, to forests, to ocean, to sky.

Many of the occupational roles filled in the natural environment allow the participant to experience something not attainable in everyday life. The challenge and imperatives of height and visual panorama, the imperative of bartering and flowing while on white water, and the scuba diver suspended in the water all involve a multi-sensory experience and provide a different perspective on reality.

In addition, inherent risks are part of the occupation. Will the rock fall, will the boat capsize, will one's knowledge and skill be sufficient to meet the demands of the occupation? In many outdoor activities, the stakes are high, and the nature of the activity forces the participant to rely upon himself or herself. Because these activities are based in the natural environment, there is a dearth of technology and mechanization. As a result, successful confrontation of the risk may enable the participant to become more secure in his or her identity and more confident in himself or herself.

The nature of outdoor risk activities demands of the participant a level of comfort with risk, uncertainty, novelty, and variety. Mountaineering, downhill racing, and hang gliding are examples of activities that possess these characteristics. The recognition of these risks varies with the experience of the participant. Through participation in the activity, skills and abilities are refined. What once seemed risky because of unmatched skills of the participant and requirements of the activity changes over the number of periods of engagement. Outfitters frequently understand this and magnify the participant's perception of risk. For example, the commercial river guide preparing a group of first-time riders "talks up" the upcoming ride. He or she orients the riders to the thrills to expect, "how the one coming up is 'a real dandy,' lost three people there last time; water's real bad now—too many rocks, don't know ... don't know ...'" (Schreyer, White, & McCool, 1980, p. 26). Next, the guide pulls off just above the rapids to "look them over," returning to strap everything securely to the raft. He or she tightens his or her life jacket. All of these behaviors, while addressing the requirements of the activity, serve to heighten the riders' sense of anticipation, fear, and excitement. Finally, the guide pushes the raft off to successfully and safely run the rapids. The riders emerge at the other end, triumphant in overcoming the river and agreeing that this is the best thing they have ever done (Schreyer et al., 1980).

Occupations that provide an escape from routine provide novelty. Unlike the everyday world, activities are less structured by mechanical time and less predictable. Successful management of the novelty and risks may result in emotional release. Activities involving risk require full concentration of attention on the task at hand—diversion can mean injury or death. This may differ for the novice and the expert in the challenges they offer. The novice may experience a release of tension as he or she completes the activity, successfully defying the dangers perceived. The expert may be more focused upon the aspects of skill and sensory arousal (Schreyer et al., 1980).

The lack of access of people with disabilities to risk-oriented, outdoor recreation activities or their avoidance of these activities may also serve to enhance the status of those with access. Until recently, few individuals with disabilities participated in adventure activities, such as hunting, climbing, kayaking, or wilderness camping. The stigma surrounding the individual with a disability as unable and incompetent fostered this lack of participation. The technological advancements in outdoor equipment, prosthetic devices, and alternative forms of mobility have increased the accessibility for participants with disabilities. Physical access, including parking lots, bathrooms, picnic areas, boat ramps, and hiking trails, continues to be upgraded to allow individuals with alternative mobility needs an opportunity to get into the natural environment.

Part of the inherent nature of occupations done outdoors is the environment itself, where humans have little control. Two obvious explanations are its sheer size and its variation from the everyday, manmade environment. In confronting this environment, one becomes knowledgeable of one's mortality and limitations that can lead to a sense of solidarity with the world, of oneness with all nature. Occupations in the outdoors involve doing something, not just listening or cognitively processing. Gone is the familiar environment with its symbols of success.

The natural environment has for centuries presented a challenge to subdue or tame it. Success and achievement in outdoor activities perhaps is symbolic of one's conquering "the Giant," a replay of David and Goliath. In contrast, lack of access to these occupations may further elevate the status of those people who do participate.

Many of our American heroes have been the cowboy, the explorer, and the overland immigrant. This is more than adequately represented in our folklore, songs, movies, and television programming. Outdoor programs provide the opportunity for participation in some of the inherent adventures portrayed in the media, thereby combining fantasy with reality.

High Adventure Activities

Activities labeled as "high adventure" focus on those outdoor activities that carry with them an inherent element of risk. They are offered through organized programs, such as Outward Bound and the National Outdoor Leadership School, which are exclusively oriented to high adventure programming. Activities include mountaineering, rafting, scuba diving, and incentive courses. Activities may be nested within a program sponsored by parks and recreation departments, university student services, and summer camps. Individuals may also engage in these activities independently of organized programs.

One characteristic of many of these activities is the sense of self-centeredness. While other members of a group can shout encouragement, it is the individual who must climb the rock face or rappel down the 200-foot drop. Unlike other activities such as football, in which the individual's performance can be enhanced or diminished by the other team members, the success or failure of the scuba diver rests on himself or herself. Risk-oriented activities require the participant to be active.

In addition, most of these activities, once initiated, must be completed. When the participant jumps feet first off the head wall, the rappel is in progress. Short of being dragged back up, the individual must complete the task. Even more obvious is the white water kayaking experience. Once the bow of the kayak enters the white water, the forces of the water require managing the rapids. A cliff jumper from California stated, "I feel it here in that compressed moment when I've crossed a line and I can't turn back. It's an intense, total commitment, a life expression" (Smith, 1998, p. D10).

Another characteristic is the high element of risk involved. The risks are multifaceted and include challenges to physical skills, psychological coping mechanisms, endurance, and problem solving. For many, successful management of the risk provides the ultimate symbol, the achievement of success in the face of fear—the defiance of death itself.

Outward Bound has become a symbol of the outdoor adventure movement. While it recognizes the nature of self-centeredness inherent to many of the adventure-based activities, the program focuses on individual learning within a group-based, collaborative effort. Instructors serve as facilitators, encouraging participants to solve problems as a group. This could be successfully negotiating a rope course or climbing wall or the completion of the daily endurance run. After all of the focus on group-based experiential learning, each participant completes a "solo." This provides both a sharp contrast to the collaborative efforts leading up to it and the opportunity for the participant to reflect upon his or her life. The solo also provides the student with the opportunity to become more sensitized to nature and to ponder his or her relationship to nature.

In stressing simplicity, informal dress is part of the expectation. Meals are shared experiences, symbolizing the communal nature of the program. Competitive rewards, such as a prize for running the fastest or cooking the best meal, common in other organized programs, do not exist in Outward Bound. Through meeting a set of challenges together over a period of time, building in opportunities to share personal reflections of the adventure experience through storytelling and journaling, Outward Bound fosters a "shared understanding" of the experience.

HUNTING

As an outdoor activity, hunting probably is one of the most controversial. Individuals object on moral grounds, and hunters counter with arguments regarding the nature of man and his role in managing the biotic community. Ortega y Gasset vividly describes hunting in the following passage:

> *The overpowering of the game, the tactile drama of its actual capture, and usually even more the tragedy of its death nurture the hunter's interest through anticipation and give liveliness and authenticity to all the previous work: the harsh confrontation with the animal's fierceness, the struggle with its energetic defense, the point of orgiastic intoxication aroused by the sight of blood, and even the hint of criminal suspicion which cross the hunter's conscience.* (1995, p. 337)

One kills in order to have hunted. The hunter seeks to conquer his or her prey through his or her own effort and skill. This involves an understanding that man is superior to the animal due to the refinement of hunting technology. The hunter may or may not attempt to give the animal a handicap in order to place man and animal on a similar level.

Yet, the killing of the animal, the goal of the hunt, symbolizes achievement, overcoming nature, and the demonstration of masculine skills. In many regions of the United States, the blood of the hunter's first kill is drunk as part of the ritual surrounding the dressing of the game. This was the custom in tribal societies as well. This symbolizes man's connection with the wild animal and may serve to both recognize and honor man's roots as a fellow animal.

In primal societies, hunting was a group phenomenon, not a solo activity. While today's hunter may go out with a group of friends to engage in the hunt, it is essentially each man against the prey. In contrast, in primitive societies, there was a clearly developed strategy with defined roles to encourage a successful hunt.

Hunting provides an acceptable way to step outside of an orderly, industrialized society. It is a socially acceptable way of expressing violence, aggression, and hostility. Because it is still an activity carried on primarily by men, it serves as a symbol of the violence and aggression "inherent in a patriarchal culture" (King, 1995, p. 358). Many would suggest that most of the acts of hunting further symbolize the domination of the male over the female. For example, the "spear's interpenetration of the animal's body is seen as 'the source of all new life'" (King, 1995, p. 368), and the symbolic relationship of male penetration into female cavities is prevalent in the description of hunters relating the kill or the field dressing of the prey.

Hunting also serves to return the hunter to his or her hunter-gatherer roots. It provides hints of a culture that saw aristocracy and nobles engaged in the hunt. For some, it may symbolize escape from work (as seen within the understanding of paid work in 20th-century America). Shepard eloquently describes how hunting returns human beings to themselves in the following:

> *The cynegetic [hunting] life is authentic because it is close to the philosophical center of human life. It constantly contrasts two central mysteries: the nature of the animal and of death. These are brought together in hunting. All other ways of life weakly confront the wild or are designed to avoid it altogether. (1973, p. 146)*

Hunting viewed within the context of American society is different from hunting done in areas where it is a requirement of survival. In the United States, most hunting is done as a form of sport or outdoor recreation and is completed for the pleasure of the hunter. While there are some arguments presented regarding the need to adequately manage wildlife numbers through hunting or the benefits to the state in revenues produced from hunting, hunting ultimately is reduced to the confrontation between man and prey. It speaks of domination of one over another. Because of this, hunting clubs, hunting preserves, commercial duck blinds, and highly sophisticated guns and bows reduce hunting to this symbol of man's superiority over nature.

FLY FISHING

The first recorded history of fly fishing was by the Greek Claudius Aelianus in 200 AD. The flies described in this document were probably more like the feathered jigs in use today. In 1496, Dame Juliana Berner published *A Treatyse of Fyshynge Wyth an Angle*. Modern fly fishing is attributed to the British who originated fly fishing as we know it. While fly fishing used to mean trying to hook a trout, it has now expanded to include fishing for many species of fresh and salt water fish.

Like many occupations, fly fishing has a language of its own. Dry flies, wet flies, streamers, nymphs, and adults all refer to types of flies. Commonly tied from a variety of natural and synthetic materials, the flies are meant to represent the natural food of the fish being sought. Fly tying in and of itself has become a reputable hobby.

The act of fly fishing requires rod, reel, line, fly, and a variety of other accessories. Formerly available only at specialty shops, a "complete fly fishing kit" can now be purchased at discount stores such as Walmart.

Those who fly fish frequently describe the occupation poetically. Part of this poetry involves the connection with the natural world in which the occupation occurs. The river, which is seen symbolically as the life stream, the sounds of the water "speaking" to the fisherman or woman, and the fish itself with its attributes of wisdom all serve to represent man's life on earth. The fish acquired these attributes in many ways. For some, the success of the fish in adapting to various habitats represents strength and adaptability. Its ability to seemingly hide, to use the streams and waterways as a way to elude man, gives it powers of intelligence. The fact that it lives in water leads humans to believe it is a clean animal. Lastly, the association with Christianity and the feeding of the thousands focuses upon its role in nurturance. The Greek letters of five Greek words form the word fish (icthys). These letters were used to stand for Jesus Christ, Son of God, Savior.

In an excerpt from his poem *Leviathian*, Conradie (1998) describes his approach to a fishing encounter:

> *Early morning frost clinging to my wading boots,*
> *I stand in a canyon, surrounded by red-brown rock,*
> *I am alone, utterly alone, with only the cry of a*
> *baboon, on the rock face somewhere high above,*
> *and the inner whisper of my being to guide me.*
>
> *I stand amidst the green of early spring, the water,*
> *crystal clear, speaks to me softly and gentle,*
> *as always.*
>
> *I listen without concentration, and hear the rambles*
> *of an old wise man, that is the river.*

Fly fishermen and women also assemble a unique wardrobe with vests of many pockets, waders, and, of course, a hat. Like other special garments, they serve to signal a belonging, a differentiation, "I am a fly fisherman." These all enable the fisherman or woman to be prepared in an instant with different flies, reels, and lines that will match the opportunity. A symbol of control and efficiency, the wardrobe also signals to others that "I am a fly fisherman."

The movie *The River Runs Through It* brought a resurged interest in fly fishing. Its representative plot of fly fishing as a metaphor for life is reiterated by Kanamoto (1998) in the following:

> *Fly fishing is, for me, a metaphor for life itself. You set for yourself a code of conduct—upstream, dry fly only, to rising trout if you are a strict moralist. You resist temptation when the fish are feeding subsurface, or you may "sin" and fish to the nymphing trout, resolving next time do better.* (1998, p. 1)

Many fly fishermen and women comment about time in discussing fly fishing. They describe the occupation as linking them to great fishers of the past, such as Halfor, Skues, and Walton—or even to the fishers of the Bible. Using the benefits of the knowledge of those past fishermen allows today's fly fishermen and women to adapt and create new traditions and rituals.

Like hunting, there is a predatory instinct to fly fishing. It requires an extensive knowledge of the natural world, of fish feeding cycles, and of the currents and eddies of the stream. Again, Kanamoto describes his sport:

> *It is a challenge, to fish with the fly. There is the thrill of stalking a truly large fish, the anticipation of the cast, the suspense of the drift, and the subsequent elation at a hook up or disappointment at the rejection. There is the adrenaline rush of the fight and the satisfaction of the catch. You can act as God and give the fish back his freedom and life, or you can exercise your ultimate right as a predator and kill him for the table.* (p. 1)

Fly fishing is considered to be an elite sport, a status symbol, due to the difficult techniques the fisherman or woman is required to master. These take time, patience, and practice to develop. Requiring rhythm and coordination, the combination of knowledge and skills creates a smoothness of effort that is both beautiful to watch and that absorbs the fishermen in its action.

SURFING

An early "extreme" sport, surfing was seen as the existential version of the modern American cowboy. Popularized in California, surfing became a way of life and a symbol of an attitude toward life. Music, hairstyles, clothing, and a party attitude represented the ultimate rejection of the American work ethic.

Surfing requires skills including upper body strength (for paddling) and balance along with a knowledge of water and wave action. In contrast to kayaking and canoeing in which the participant skims above the water, the surfer is in the wave. The surfer engages in his or her sport in an upright position; he or she becomes a water walker! Until recently, surfing was taught in a manner much like the apprenticing of craftsmen. Expert surfers taught novices, and an oral tradition of surfing education fostered. More recently, surf schools have become more dominant, especially in California and Hawaii. This has created some tension between those who consider themselves "surfers" and the beginners.

Newman (1998) describes the feeling of surfing in the following excerpt from his article:

You are out on the wave, sunning yourself like a sea turtle on the deck of your long board, buoyantly contemplating the various forces of the universe that have brought you to this point in your life, to this peculiarly exhilarating moment. Then, in an instant, three-fourths of the earth's surface erupts into a wall beneath you, propelling you relentlessly ahead on the architecture of speed and possibility. (p. D15)

GARDENING

Horticulture has been described as the interaction of a person with the plant world. This can occur through a person actively working with plants, passively viewing plants, or creating craft products from plant materials. Gardening is one aspect of horticulture. Gardening implies action. This action may involve doing things with plants or to plants to enhance or modify their growth. This active engagement in the life cycle of plants is seen as a euphemism and symbol of the act of birth and nurturing, Mother Nature again!

Plants provide an understanding of the cyclic nature of life. Seeing a plant throughout its lifespan from seed, to plant, to withered stalk creates a natural symbol for the life process of humans. Stirrup (1998) explains,

When I first grew lettuce I let many of the plants bolt, flower, and go to seed. I wanted to see what lettuce looked like in all its stages, not just what I saw in the supermarket. It was a surprising and humbling experience. (p. 1)

Gardening also provides a vivid contrast to what Stirrup describes as people's expectations of one peak life experience after another. The media portray life as full of laughing, smiling people—ecstatic over their new cars, cold beer, and shiny hair. They lead the viewer to expect a life of "highs." When that doesn't happen, they become frustrated or depressed. Gardening keeps gardeners in the moment. Plants reveal the truth in concrete ways, unable to pretend everything is okay. When they need water, they wilt. When they are cared for, observed, watered, and fed, they frequently flourish. Certainly a metaphor for the social existence of humans.

Relf (1981) describes a number of ways that specific forms of gardening may be symbolic to the gardener. The staking of a tomato plant may symbolize to the gardener that other living things need support, that the gardener can be useful to another living thing by providing that support. Through this, the gardener comes to see that he or she is worthwhile and can aid another who "cannot stand alone" (p. 3). Unlike human interaction, plants do this in a nonthreatening and nondiscriminatory manner.

McQueen (as cited in Rossbach, 1991) describes how he views the gardener's work with trees being both a symbol for nature and for man's need to control nature:

> *I think we see trees as a symbol of nature, both good and bad. We feel we have to control them, prune them, and thin them out. I'm sure they'd be perfectly happy without that. It's our way of being in charge of the world, and I think a tree stands for that ....* (p. 15-16)

In urban communities, the need of humans to prune, shape, and protect the trees supersedes. They are pruned and shaped just as humans are to meet the expectations of society.

Choices of plants for one's garden can become symbols of one's own individuality. Orchids may be chosen because they are rare, expensive, and difficult to grow—thereby becoming a status symbol. They are a symbol of beauty or indulgence. Vegetables may be chosen because of an urge to return to one's agrarian roots, to be able to provide sustenance and exist more independently. Organic gardening offers the opportunity to both redirect man's desire to control and overpower nature while at the same time offering a perceived healthier lifestyle. The organic gardener frequently desires a return to a simpler, more holistic life, and the garden becomes a tangible signal for this life.

Gardening also has a component of passive participation. Walking in the woods and admiring the trees, looking at a floral arrangement, or enjoying the landscape during a rain storm all are essentially passive in regards to the occupation of gardening. Many view parts of the plant kingdom as being especially meaningful as McQueen (as cited in Rossbach, 1991) explains,

> *Trees represent the accumulation of our concept of nature stored in our unconscious ... they are an image of our fear of nature; a fairy tale fear of the "deep, dark woods" where man is lost and out of his element.* (p. 15)

Flowers have been used as major symbols in the work of artists such as Georgia O'Keefe and Salvador Dali. They are integral to the rituals surrounding birth, death, and marriage. For example, sending flowers upon the death of someone serves symbolic purposes. The flowers are a symbol of love, caring, and concern. They also serve to brighten the atmosphere and serve as a diversion.

The use of flowers and plants as both a symbol and a method of communication began in Constantinople in the 1600s. It was brought to England in 1716 by Lady Mary Wortley Montagu. In Victorian England, flowers became a way for lovers to communicate without the knowledge of their chaperones. Flowers and floral arrangements served to make simple statements and to convey complex messages. For example, daisies were viewed as symbols of love and innocence, carnations as a symbol of "I'll never forget you," crocuses as a symbol of cheerfulness, and poppies as a symbol of eternal sleep. The corn poppy came to symbolize remembrance of those who died in the war. The manner in which flowers were exchanged also served as a message. Presented upright they contained a positive meaning, upside down they were meant to convey the opposite meaning. Many of these meanings and customs continue today.

Plants have also developed hidden meanings. The laurel represents achievement; myrtle represents love; and ivy represents fidelity. Straw has come to symbolize agreement, while witch hazel indicates a spell. Woven together into a wreath, plants and flowers symbolize eternity. They served in ancient times as the link between the dead and his or her life forces. The Egyptian word *ankh* means both wreath and wood. When conversation arises that brings foreboding, the individual will do or say, "touch wood." This arose from the belief that plants and trees gave protection against evil forces.

Living plants were also seen as a cleansing vehicle. The plants or wreath came to represent the vital force of the plants and was used both to cleanse and remove guilt. The material of the wreath also carried their own symbols. At weddings, the bride and groom wore wreaths made of quince leaves (sacred to Juno, the goddess of marriage) and marjoram (associated with Hymen, the wedding god).

Later wreaths were associated with winners of athletic contests and war. Most frequently used plants were the olive tree (Olympics) and laurel (the Pythian Games at Delphi). Laurel wreaths were expanded in use and came to symbolize the poet and musician. Wreaths were worn by royalty and used by Christians. Roman soldiers were said to have mocked Jesus, placing a wreath or crown of thorns on his head to symbolize "King of the Jews."

CAMPING

Camping requires individuals to live in the outdoors. This may be in an environment that closely simulates home, like a motor home or trailer, or it may be under canvas or under the stars. Many believe that the appeal of camping lies in an attempt to emulate the early nomadic lifestyle of humankind, or it may represent the early settlers in the United States and their gradual moving, with the frontier, westward. Camping also provides an alternative to expensive lodging, such as condominiums, cabins, and motels. For some, it serves as a symbol of rebellion against the materialism these others types of lodging represent.

Like other activities done in the outdoors, camping immerses the camper in his or her environment. It is a sensory experience. The smell of the campfire, feel of the hard ground, taste of s'mores or banana boats, sound of the owls in the tree, and sight of the sun setting over the campsite arouse the senses of the participant. Each person reacts to this input dependent on his or her experience.

Some types of camping require the camper to "rough it." These provide an escape from organized, urban life. They require more self-reliance. For example, backpacking requires the camper to carry the "campsite" on the back. The location of the campsite is in the wilderness where the camper may have to construct a toilet, erect the tent, and develop a makeshift kitchen. This contributes to a sense of self-reliance.

The type of shelter frequently symbolizes the camper's personal philosophy toward nature. The backpacker, carrying the campsite on the back, becomes the nomad of old. In close touch with nature, the floor of the forest becomes the bed. Bathing occurs in streams and lakes. The outdoors offers a novel environment in which to briefly live. In contrast to backpacking, campgrounds provide a social atmosphere away from the expectations of business. The size of the trailer, motor home, or pop-up camper and its amenities are status symbols against which other campers compare themselves.

The campsite also serves as a staging area for a number of other activities associated with camping, such as hiking, climbing, boating, fishing, and bird watching. Within the site, other social events take place. These may include songs around the campfire, sharing meals, card games, and storytelling. Hunting and foraging activities, often gender segregated, reinforce male and female roles and images. Around the campsite, women may still be the primary cooks, while men chop the wood. These reflect differing lifestyles and values.

More than any other part of camping, the campfire seems to be remembered the longest. It provides more of a contrast to the urban environment than anything else. Whether it is enjoyed as part of an organized camp or while camping alone or with friends, the fire offers warmth and comfort. Rituals are part of the campfire. This may be a song or a favorite method of lighting the fire. In organized camps, the fire is lit using traditional means, such as flint and steel or a flaming torch. It is frequently lit while kneeling. This symbolizes man's respect for fire and his acknowledgement of its role in survival. Campfires occur at night, offering a respite to the day's activities. They represent a time to relax and reflect. The fire serves to provide light against the darkness and to create a safe haven in which to rest.

Nature's Challenge

This chapter has presented some ideas regarding the codes of meaning associated with nature's challenges. Representative activities served as examples of the unique symbolism associated with activities that use the outdoors as an inherent part of the activity. Other chapters have discussed alternative occupations chosen by individuals. Earlier in this book, you completed a set of questions regarding your secondary occupations. To better understand the variety of meanings associated with these occupations, find someone to interview regarding his or her secondary occupation. What are the similarities and differences between your activity profile and his or hers. What relationship does this have to life satisfaction and quality of life?

Think about the following questions on Page 91. Identify your responses to the interviewer after each question. Reflect upon your responses and describe your repertoire of secondary occupations to this point in your life.

1. Briefly describe your current hobbies and activity interests.

2. How would you categorize each in relation to the following qualities?

Active _____Passive

Participant_____Observer

Competitive _____Cooperative

Gross Motor Skills _____Fine Motor Skills

Free Expression _____Structure

High Level of Cognitive _____Low Level of Cognitive

Skill Required   Skill Required

High Degree of Social _____Low Degree of Social

or Cultural Relevance   or Cultural Relevance

High Interpersonal/ _____Low Interpersonal/

Social Level   Social Level

3. What motivates you to be involved in these hobbies/activities?

4. Which is/are your favorite(s)? What aspects make each special?

5. How frequently are you involved in each?

6. What factors limit your involvement? What factors enhance your involvement?

7. How are these similar/different from your childhood activities? How are these similar/different from your primary occupation?

8. On the basis of the above, how would you characterize your activity profile?

REFERENCES

Conradie, J. (1998, August 5). *Leviathian*. http://www.uky.edu/-agrdanny/flyfish/muse/conradie.htm.

Kanamoto, H. (1998, August 5). *Why I flyfish*. http://www.uky.edu/-agrdanny/flyfish/muse/kanamoto.htm.

King, R. J. H. (1995). Environmental ethics and the case against hunting. In: W. J. Morgan & K. V. Meier (Eds.). *Philosophic inquiry in sport,* 2nd ed. (pp. 357-372). Champaign, IL: Human Kinetics.

Merchant, C. (1998). The death of nature. In: M. E. Zimmerman, J. B. Callicott, G. Sessions, K. J. Warren, & J. Clark (Eds.). *Environmental philosophy*, 2nd ed. (pp. 277-290). Upper Saddle River, NJ: Prentice Hall.

Newman, B. (1998, March 11). Her dog can surf, all right, but what about her students? *The New York Times*.

Ortega y Gasset, J. (1995). The ethics of hunting. In: W. J. Morgan & K. V. Meier (Eds.). *Philosophic inquiry in sport*, 2nd ed. (pp. 334-338). Champaign, IL: Human Kinetics.

Relf, D. (1981). Dynamics of horticulture therapy. *Rehabilitation Literature, 42,* 147-150.

Rossbach, E. (1991) Containment and being contained. In: V. Halper & E. Rossbach (Eds.). *John McQueen: The language of containment* (pp. 13-24). Washington, DC: Smithsonian Institution.

Schreyer, R. M., White, R., & McCool, S. F. (1980). Common attributes uncommonly exercised. In: J. F. Meier, T. W. Morash, & G. E. Welton (Eds.). *High adventure outdoor pursuits: Organization and leadership* (pp. 24-29). Columbus, OH: Publishing Horizons, Inc.

Shepard, P. (1973). *The tender carnivore and the sacred game*. New York: Scribners.

Smith, C. (1998, March 11). Moab's natives struggle with an overabundance of wildlife. *The New York Times*.

Stirrup, M. (1998, August 5). *The garden as teacher*. http://www.icangarden.com/featartc.htm.

ADDITIONAL READING

Regen, T. (1995). Why hunting and trapping are wrong. In: W. J. Morgan & K. V. Meier (Eds.). *Philosophic inquiry in sport*, 2nd ed. (pp. 347-350). Champaign, IL: Human Kinetics.

Weber, B. (1998, March 11). The thrill of risk, and other reasons why. *The New York Times*.

The Language of Crafts

Beth P. Velde

Crafts are distinguished from the fine arts covered later in this book in that they are the celebration of everyday life. They serve to link the past and present and help to bind one individual to another through the creation of a product. This distinction is arbitrary and somewhat artificial, for art and craft overlap each other. However, for the sake of this discussion, craft will refer to those things that use materials for decorative, useful, or manipulative purposes and are made from a variety of substances. They are linked to manual dexterity, attention to detail, and skill.

Crafts are functional. In the creation of the craft, it is their ultimate use that demands a certain form and makes it recognizable. A vessel meant to hold water must have a certain shape and a particular opening to facilitate pouring. It is functional when the shape works well for the purpose it was created. It is recognizable to its users because of its shape and size and is distinguishable from a vessel meant to hold olive oil or cream because of its configuration. While it may be considered beautiful by others, the beauty does not detract from its function. Yanagi (as cited in Shaw, 1993) explains,

> *Utility does not permit unsoundness or frailty, for between use and beauty there is a close relationship. Utility demands faithfulness in objects; it does not condone human self-indulgence. In creating an object intended for practical use, the maker does not push himself to the foreground or even, for that matter, to the surface.* (p. 8)

Crafts have a long and rich history in humankind. Before the advent of toolmaking, hunter-gatherers used their own hands to survive. Men brought home the hides of animals, which women prepared for use as shelter, clothing, and food containers. With the advent of tools and metal, men began to take over some of the crafts. In addition to use in everyday survival, they crafted objects of war. Early crafts used the natural materials easily found in the environment, such as reeds, clay, and animal by-products. The production and refinement of crafts was a demonstration of human problem-solving abilities. Flint knives were fashioned to make cutting easier. Pounding tools were created to make flattening materials easier. Eventually, new materials were used to create products and material for craft products.

Crafts are carried on through a tradition of craft making that is encouraged and taught by community and family members to each other. Frequently, the crafts reflect a cultural system that may consist of a family group, age group, ethnic group, religious group, or work-related group. For example, a family group may pass on the custom of creating an elaborate picture album describing family history and communicating family values. Ukrainian groups may teach the craft of Pysanky, or Ukrainian Easter egg painting. Community groups may get together to create an AIDS quilt, or groups of battered/abused women may develop T-shirts representing their experience to be hung in the Clothesline Project. Women's groups at the local church may sew the elaborate banners used to decorate the altars during religious events. Sailors share rituals and crafts associated with marine life, and the creation of elaborate knotted macramé hangings are based on the knots the sailors use during the work day. Scrim shaw is an excellent example of sailor craft, which is highly artistic in nature.

In early America, three different craft groups existed. *Professional tradespeople*, such as blacksmiths and cabinet makers, were trained in apprenticeship programs. *Itinerant craftspeople* did not receive as structured a training. They learned the crafts from each other in a loosely structured network and completed their crafts for both pleasure and to produce a modest profit. These were the weavers, potters, basket makers, and tinsmiths. The *homes craftspeople* primarily learned from family and used their products to embellish their own homes (Shaw, 1993).

What is the meaning behind crafts? For many, it represents a way to exert some control over their lives. It is a chance to prove that one can exist without the machine-made goods to which we have grown accustomed. Crafts also allow the creator to leave little bits of himself or herself in the end product, the product becoming a manifestation of self. The role of crafter further allows the individual to assume the role of artist, raising his or her status and role within a given society. This is especially true when the crafts are sold and become a profit-making enterprise. In a society where crafts are acknowledged, the master craftsperson becomes a valued person within the society. This role is important, because crafts are often taught by one person to another.

The outcome of the craft experience is a tangible object. Often, this object is useful in some aspect of everyday life and may also serve to enhance the beauty of the environment. Many authors further suggest that crafts serve as a metaphor for life. The crafter "receives basic raw materials, and through a series of efforts, waiting periods and guidance, one lives a life—and creates a craft product" (Drake, 1992, p. 4).

The end product of crafts may be given to others, a way to "pay back" another's support, friendship, or even services. Sometimes, they serve as a means to occupy one's time or to keep one's mind off other matters while still being productive. Hence, because the crafter is creating something and occupying his or her hands, literally and figuratively he or she is not "wasting" time.

Craft products provide the owner with the opportunity to surround himself or herself with customs and objects that sustain him or her. As tangible signs of oneself and one's heritage, they offer familiar aspects of a cultural and personal continuum that bring comfort to the owner. Scrapbooking is one such example. Individuals engaged in this craft create elaborate albums of photographs and personal mementos that display one's life story. Scrapbooks are a way of cementing oneself in history. They provide a sense of identity and create a social history. Armed with photographs, textured and colored paper, die cuts, stickers, hole punches and scissors, groups of scrapbookers gather together in settings reminiscent of the quilting bees of old. Sharing ideas, personal stories, and supplies, they create elaborate personal narratives.

When compared to each other, some are more adaptable and responsive, allowing for mistakes. When working in clay, it is possible to create, destroy, and create again from the same raw materials. Crafts also allow for creativity, the contribution of something uniquely mine to the world around me. According to Tillman (1973), "A person can be creative and do imitative work; the original person invents deviations from the known and expected" (p. 155).

In the process of creation, the craft requires the crafter to become intimately engaged with the materials. The moistness and pliability of the clay in potting, the sharpness of the needle in quilting, the odor of the liver of sulfur in copper tooling all place demands on the individual that are multisensory in nature. These sensual experiences create a contrast to the everyday life of many people's existence. This involvement also sensitizes the crafter to the effort involved in creation. While the same object may be purchased cheaper due to mass production, it may have less value to the crafter because of the lack of contribution of the individual.

Like the arbitrary distinction between art and craft, crafts themselves are divided into categories for the purposes of discussion. Some are based upon the material used: wood, paper, fiber, reeds, or metal. A second perspective is to focus on the process, hence, pottery, sewing, painting, leatherwork, woodworking, or weaving. Finally, they may be based upon the purpose of the action in the craft: expressive crafts, image crafts, kinetic crafts, instrumental crafts, utilitarian crafts, decorative crafts, sale crafts, or learning crafts. This categorization expresses something about both the actions and purposes of the action processes. Using categorical divisions for crafts often fulfills a need for program planners and marketers. The categories also help us to focus on different aspects of the crafts in terms of their meaning. When addressing the approach of the types of materials to define a category, one can better understand the activities' meaning through the characteristics of the materials. Hence, clay with its pliability and adaptability may be seen symbolically as the raw material of one's life. The ability to create, destroy, and create again from the same lump of clay can serve as a metaphor for living.

In grouping crafts by the process used, one can perceive the craft in relationship to one's daily actions. Weaving can be seen as the creation of one's personal narrative, combining the warp (one's personal history and innate skills and abilities) with the weft (the interaction that occurs on a daily basis with the world around one). If one were to combine this approach with the first, the materials used in the weaving would add to the symbolism. Reeds are a type of material that are difficult to work with, being rigid and less flexible. Yarn, on the other hand, is softer to the touch, more pliable, and easier to cut and shape. The combination of the process with the material creates a different metaphor.

Lastly, the purpose of the action focuses on the role of the participant. A weaving completed as a product of personal expression, in which both creativity and originality may be the focus, has a different meaning than one completed for strictly utilitarian purposes.

A number of crafts tend to be viewed in our western world as gender oriented. Those that have traditionally been used primarily by women are sewing, embroidery, or textile painting. Those most frequently associated with men are woodworking, metal hammering, or leatherwork.

The economic value of a craft is influenced by durability, availability of the craft material, and production processes. Real leather versus vinyl, oak versus pine, or gold compared to silver are all more costly and valued more by their owners. Crafts may gain symbolic meaning based on their durability. Mosaics and ceramics are more durable than baskets.

The world of crafts is filled with symbols represented in the objects created as well as in the materials and tools used in the making. The actions and processes involved in creating, in making the crafts, are replete with symbolic and inferred messages. The hammering of tinsmithing and wedging of pottery may be cathartic tools for the release of aggression or frustration. The natural desire of humans to shape, smear, feel, squeeze, and mold are released in such craft materials as clay. Here, there is effort needed to control the clay, especially in comparison to other crafts in which structure is imposed. There is symbolic meaning in the making and destruction of clay objects.

Crafts vary in the level and type of social interaction required. Sewing can be a solitary or extra-individual activity, requiring only the interaction of a person with an object. In contrast, it can be a collaborative or intragroup activity as in quilting, in which a set of craftspeople come together to share an experience, collaborate on the production of a quilt, and illustrate a historical tradition. Crafts can be multilateral in nature, where there is competition among three or more people, with no one person as an antagonist. An example of this would be a judged event, such as a county fair where awards are given to craft products in selected categories. A typical craft shop is an example of aggregate social interaction in which action is directed by the individual toward an object while in the company of others. However, there is no interaction required between participants; everyone is working on his or her own project. Avedon (1971) provides a more complete description of the requirements of social interaction inherent in activities.

Many occupations involve crafts. These include nature-oriented activities, camping, dramatics, dance, music, and social activities. For example, crafts are frequently used to illustrate parts of a drama. Costumes are constructed, and sets are designed. They may also be part of a creation of the objects used in the drama, for example puppets. In nature-oriented activities, individuals may create useful objects, such as lashed tables, shelters of canvas or wood, water vehicles, such as canoes, or spoons of whittled wood.

Sorensen (1992) suggests that crafts provide individuals with direct experience with materials that can be translated into larger messages about life:

You analogize the skills to everyday circumstances, such as how to use pressure (when you push too hard, you wreck it); how to deal with resistance (work steadily around it); when to be gentle and when to be forceful (you can control it); and when to stop, rest, or work it (you'll get tired and smear it, or the media has to dry) ... learning to master what I see and touch can help me to master what I think and feel.

CRAFT CONSTRUCTIONS

The process of creating an end product involves interaction of the crafter with both the environment and the craft materials. This may occur in a highly structured nature as in following a dress pattern or pouring a ceramic mold or a less structured fashion as in sculpting with clay. Crafters may also exhibit creativity by modifying an existing protocol, changing the materials used, or in combining two protocols or media. Using objects in a way they were not intended is part of this process of creation. Tin cans become elaborate lanterns or wind chimes, light bulbs become castanets, and wooden spoons become puppets.

Do crafters engage in the process solely for the production of an end product? Perhaps it is reasonable to assume that many engage in the occupation because of the process of crafting. This process involves a holistic experience in which kinesthetic demands merge with aesthetic demands. To bend a reed into a particular configuration to create a basket or to develop an idea for an actual product may facilitate a feeling of self-satisfaction. The opportunity to produce a material good where there was none before often results in self-fulfillment. Crafts may provide individuals with a way to escape the constrictions of societal rules and express an inner sense of self. Crafts achieve elements of language when the product becomes an expression of emotions, desires, and ideals visible to self and others.

CRAFTSMANSHIP

Craftsmanship is an integral part of the craft process. The quality of the end product relates to the ability of the individual to match his or her skills with the demands of the craft. Those that are done well come from the investment of an individual in both the process and the completion of the end product. Often, the quality is judged by the person producing it. Crafts that are poorly done are those that are done hastily, without attention to the detail and processes necessary to complete the project. It is unrealistic to expect that quality is not also judged against another's end product. This is especially relevant in sales crafts. However, craftsmanship results in pride. It is a product of the time invested. The piece of handiwork carries the reputation of the producer.

Crafts involve engagement in a production process from start to finish. Many commercially made products are a result of an assembly line. Workers do pieces of the production, but no one person is invested in every step. Because of this, time is inextricably linked to crafting. In machine-made goods, quantity produced and time required are measures of productivity. In handmade crafts, the crafter becomes uniquely aware of time. The process of crafting encourages focus, meditation, a manipulation of time against other demands, and finally an appreciation of time relative to the product. Most crafters modularize time to allow for the process of crafting amidst other responsibilities. But time must be managed relative to the product. Sometimes, the product demands that a sequence be completed; it cannot be broken up for the sake of mechanical time. This forces its maker to recognize his or her inability to be totally in control of time and enhances his or her appreciation for the rhythmicity of time not controlled by an arbitrary device such as a clock. In a phenomenological sense, the craftsman and the craft cannot be separated.

TOOLS OF THE CRAFTER

Over time, the tools used in crafts have acquired symbolic meaning. The hammer was the tool used in many craft and work sites. Its association in this way has resulted in the hammer viewed as a symbol for work. Another tool widely associated with both work and craft is the knife. Carvers, tanners, shoemakers, woodsmen, hunters, gardeners, cooks, and fishermen all view the knife as indispensable. A knife with the appearance of a dagger has come to represent violence and death, and a Swiss Army knife has come to symbolize resourcefulness and mastery in one's environment. Young boys see the acquisition of a pocket knife as a rite of passage to responsibility and acceptance in a man's world.

Craft objects are viewed symbolically. The chair allows one to sit in an elevated position. The person seated is viewed as having more dignity and power than the one who is left standing. The decoration, size, form, and position of the chair may symbolize rank and social status. The rocking chair has come to symbolize comfort and nurturing as in rocking an infant to sleep. Candles, another form of craft product, are viewed symbolically as a way to dispel darkness thereby averting evil, to signify hope, and as an expression of joy. Candles are used in sacred ceremonies and signify devotion, repentance, and to represent a loved one who has died. Candles also serve as an image of human life and spirit. Bowls and jugs, whether made of clay, wood, or tin, serve as symbols themselves and for what they hold. This may have begun with offerings to the gods, many of which were of liquid form. The water jug came to symbolize the gift of life, fertility, rebirth, and eternal life (Achen, 1978).

While there is not time to cover all crafts and their potential meaning, this chapter will conclude with a discussion of Pysanky, sand painting, wood crafts, quilting, weaving, basket making, and pottery to provide examples of how the above discussion relates to specific crafts.

PYSANKY

Combining color and symbols upon an egg, the making of Pysanky a few weeks before Easter each year represents an old Ukrainian custom. Eggs are ancient symbols. In neolithic times, the egg represented the sun and its ability to give life. In the spring when the warmth of the sun's rays returned and things began to grow, people decorated eggs and distributed them during celebrations. With the onset of Christianity, the custom continued. The eggs came to symbolize Christian rebirth. The Ukrainians decorated two types of eggs, the krashanky, which were hardboiled eggs dyed bright colors and later eaten, and the Pysanky, which were decorated elaborately and kept for their decorative and symbolic purposes.

The Pysanky were believed to have special powers and were used to heal, protect the home from fire, ensure a good harvest, and bring fertility to a childless couple. Each egg is unique, and the exact design is never duplicated. The egg is created from a framework. First, the egg is divided into geometric areas of wide bands, triangles, or ovals within which further designs are made. The tools and materials include a fresh egg, candle, lump of beeswax, a kistka, and dye. The kistka, a tiny metal spout, is heated over a candle and pressed into the beeswax. The melted wax is scooped into the spout and designs are drawn on the egg. The egg is dipped into dye, where the beeswax lines resist the dye. This continues, and a number of different dyes are used. Finally, the egg is warmed until the wax melts and is wiped off, revealing the design.

Symbols used on the Pysanky reflect both issues relevant to everyday life and to spiritual life. The sun is used to represent life and growth. Eternal youth and health are symbolized through the evergreen. Other plants are used, including the flower that stands for love. Animals are also used. In keeping with the symbolism of the egg itself, the hen represents fertility, while the deer symbolizes good will and wealth. Tied to prosperity, wheat is related to good health and a bountiful harvest. Christianity is represented by a more universal symbol, the fish.

NAVAJO SAND PAINTING

Originally part of a religious ceremony to heal the sick or mentally disturbed, Navajo sand paintings have recently been preserved and are replicated by craftspeople throughout the United States. Traditionally, the Navajo believe that illness is caused by breaking taboos or in some way being out of tune with the natural world. The creation of a sand painting was used by the medicine man to bring a person back in tune with the universe. Using materials he has gathered from the environment (pollen, crushed flowers, charcoal, pulverized sandstone, and other minerals), the medicine man spreads clean sand on the floor of the hogan. Using the natural materials gathered, he allows them to sift through his fingers in designs traditional for each illness. Figures include holy people—straight-bodied figures; sacred plants such as corn, beans, squash, and tobacco; bluebirds (a symbol of happiness); and the sun, moon, rain, and lightning. These may be surrounded on the north, south, and west by a rainbow that protects the painting from evil.

As each element of the design is made, chants are sung that ask for help from the holy people. The person to be cured, the family, and friends all gather to take part in the ceremony. Because the sacred painting must never be desecrated, it is destroyed by scattering it to the four winds after the ceremony. Increasingly, this ancient ceremony is coupled with modern doctors in the treatment of the Navajo. Because of the beauty and symbolism of this craft, Navajo are creating sand painting on boards, using glue to make a permanent design. While not associated with the religious ceremony, these carry much of the symbolic meaning characteristic of the authentic sand painting (Schuman, 1981).

WOOD CRAFTS

Carving and construction using natural wood is another element of the craft genre. Selection of the wood is an important first step in the process. Many craftsmen prefer wood that is indigenous to the area because they feel it best represents the values and beliefs of the culture. Oak is well known for both its beauty and durability. It is symbolic of strength and longevity.

Many carvers view their role as setting the wood free, allowing the figures and symbols inherent in the wood to be accentuated. As part of the Philadelphia Folklore Project, Furman Humphrey was interviewed regarding his work as a carver. In discussing the process of carving, he describes how a crook in the grain may become a serpent, a knot, an animal, or face. Much of his work includes animal and human figures, which draws on his early experiences growing up in North Carolina. They illustrate in his mind "how things ought to be" (Lindsey, 1994a, p. 4). While the art of carving is representative of a folk craft, walking sticks were a necessity in many areas and were used to provide support in walking on uneven terrain, ward off animals, and clear overgrown pathways. The walking sticks "become a link to the past, to parents, the rural home community, and youth. Highly carved or otherwise ornamented canes have traditionally symbolized respect and authority in many communities" (p. 4).

QUILTING

Needlework is composed of a variety of forms including embroidery, garment construction, tapestry, quilting, and others. Unlike the pen, the needle has always been thought of as a woman's instrument. She used it to express herself in socially acceptable forms.

Quilting in the 19th century was closely associated with the preparation for marriage. Oral folk descriptions suggest that 13 quilts had to be accumulated prior to marriage, but 19th century inventories appear to support between seven and 10 as the usual number. Quilting bees frequently took place immediately before the wedding, where the final quilt was completed. "These bridal quilts became particularly treasured possessions and served as a tangible reminder of goodwill and hope for a fruitful union" (Lindsey, 1994b, p. 4). Quilting bees also provided a break from the solitary life of the frontier family, where the nearest neighbor was miles away. The quilting bee came to symbolize women working together.

Around 1840, another type of quilt became important in symbolizing the nurturance and friendship among American women. The friendship, album, or signature quilts were designs that were best known by the signature of each contributor on the block that she made. A special type of friendship quilt, the freedom quilt, was designed and given to a young man to signify his coming of age and the end of an apprenticeship where he was still under the control of both parents and craft master. These quilts carried the symbols of freedom and masculinity—eagles, ships, guns, horses, and fraternal orders (Atkins, 1994).

Traditional quilts are bed coverings made up of three layers—a backing, a center filling, and a decorative top. The layers are hand sewn together using a needle and thread. The top may be plain, pieced, and/or appliqued. America's most significant contribution to quilting was the refinement of pieced work used in creating quilt tops. The piecing together of small segments of fabric was often born of necessity as life in colonial and frontier America was stark and resources scarce. Large pieces of fabric were expensive, so scraps and recycled material became a way to save money. These pieces were cut into various shapes and sewn together to create blocks and geometric shapes. Successful pattern designs, such as log cabin, star of Bethlehem, and wedding ring, are still used today.

Quilts in these early days were made to be durable. The small pieces could be easily replaced if worn or torn. The technique of piecing was easy to learn and became a decorative art. The quality and design of a quilt became a way of recognizing the identity of the quilter and representative to some extent of the woman's worth.

They are perhaps the most visible and enduring documents of the everyday lives of 19th-century American women of every race and social class, and they represent an exuberant, expressive, and passionate parallel history of the growth of the burgeoning new country (Shaw, 1993). Quilts came to represent traditional values, in which tightly knit communities, honoring God and country, and family relationships were seen as the core to happiness.

Quilts also reflect the culture and history of a region. The Amish developed a quilting style that reflected and symbolized their lifestyle. Frequently using plain materials of subdued colors, their designs employed a limited number of controlled geometric patterns, such as center diamond, diamond-in-the-square, four-patch, nine-patch, and bars all made up of pieces cut into the three basic angled shapes of the square, triangle, or rectangle. African American quilters devised a more free and improvisational approach. Instead of primarily using stitching to combine pieces of fabric, these quilters employed brightly colored yarns tied to bind the layers of the quilt together. Today, in recognition of the time it takes to create a handcrafted quilt, quilts are used as decorative items and are hung on walls or made in smaller dimensions and used as throws.

Quilts have taken many forms in recent years. Presentation quilts continue to be made and presented to those who deserve honor and recognition. Service-oriented groups, like the Red Cross, continue to make quilts both to sell and raise money for projects and to give to those in need. Groups of like-minded individuals gather together to create a quilt to convey a message, such as the AIDS Memorial Quilt created by the NAMES Project. Quilts are unique in their ability to represent individual creativity and collaborative effort in one product. Symbolically, they may represent hope, resilience, interdependence, or serve as a metaphor for society itself.

WEAVING

Weaving is an ancient craft originating in Europe. Looms vary from the floor loom of four or eight harnesses to the Navajo loom, typically erected outside. Weavings consist of a warp over which a weft thread is intertwined to produce a variety of patterns. As thread and yarn have been refined, the visual impact of the weft has decreased with the predominant pattern carried by the weft. Anthropologists report tribal traditions in early New Guinea and other areas that involved isolating the bride-to-be away from the tribe with a loom to weave a coverlet just prior to marriage. This was used to cover the bridal bed, symbolizing the joining of warp and weft, of two parts into one.

Cloth, as an important aspect of early American households, was a woman's contribution to the community. Spinning wheels were frequently taken on a social visit, and spinning contests were common. Cloth-making was a popular entry at county fairs. Together, these served to reward a woman who was skilled at spinning and weaving and served to improve the quality of handmade cloth. The demand for cloth eventually led to the industrialization of the process, which, in turn, affected hand-weaving and other crafts dependent on cloth (such as quilting). During the American Revolution, the hand-making of cloth served as a symbol of both American pride and self-reliance, as the patriots refused to purchase imported English goods.

Weavers contributed to the success of the early American colonists, providing coverlets woven of wool and later silk. These served to protect the owner against the cold and to brighten the bedroom. The type of coverlet served as a sign of the status of the owner. The simpler to weave overshot coverlet was less costly and time-intensive to make. The double weave was afforded by the more well-to-do.

Basket Making

Basket making is a craft about construction. It frequently uses natural materials, such as reeds, grasses, and natural yarns, although man-made fibers and materials can be used. This connection to the natural world links the basket maker to natural time and natural rhythms. Materials have to be gathered at the appropriate time of the year to be usable. This creates a natural rhythm, a relationship with nature that may not exist in other crafts. McQueen (as cited in Rossbach, 1991) describes his relationship with one of the materials he prefers in the following quote:

> *I think about what a tree is, the nature of a tree, how it is organized, what it stands for. I think a basket is about organization. Our minds are always organizing things. That's one part. The other part is the mythology of trees.* (p. 14)

Baskets are also linked to the past of human civilization—perhaps one of the first crafted objects created by a human hand. Their use links the user to his or her distant ancestors. Basket making later became associated with children's summer camps, merit badges, and therapy in mental institutions. The term "basket making" began to be used in a derogatory manner, implicating non-intellectual work or busywork (Rossbach, 1986). Many of the baskets in use today are made in developing countries, where labor is cheap. They are produced quickly and sold cheaply. They become stigmatized with their methods of production—cheap labor, poverty, illiteracy, and the non-intellect (Rossbach, 1986). In contrast, in industrialized countries, baskets are being mass produced of plastic using a process of molding. In the process, they lose their connection with the natural world and with man as homo faber. Perhaps more than anything, they lose their meaning. Halper (1991) explains the symbolism of baskets:

> *... Baskets are shells that divide inner from outer space and allow the artist to ruminate on the qualities of separation and isolation that the baskets possess: Does the basket enfold or exclude? Does it suggest security or entrapment? Can the isolated object, a reductive artifact, address the complex and inclusive natural world? Can the container, a model of concision, also be a model of human thought and language?* (p. 41-42)

Pottery

Unlike basket making, in which the crafter appears in control of the product, potters seem to be more at the will of the clay with which they work. Clay has characteristics of plasticity unlike the natural materials used in basket making. Whether hand building or working on a wheel, the potter appears to be "an attentive observer while the clay moves and changes, searching for its own form, which it achieves through trial and error" (Rossbach, 1986, p. 182).

A second difference lies in the process of construction itself. While the basket maker predominantly uses his or her hands to fashion the basket, the potter becomes engaged with the clay, using his or her whole body. Whether wedging, rolling, centering on the wheel, or raising the clay form, the potter's involvement includes his or her whole body.

Pottery as an American craft is linked to the Native Americans, especially to those residing in the American Southwest. The Indian potters used hand building as opposed to the potters wheel to create their products. This resulted in pots with very thin walls, thinner than could have been achieved at the wheel. Decorations were often symbolic and abstract, usually representing natural phenomena. These included the sun, sky, rain, clouds, and various animal forms. Once decorated, they were fired in open kilns, fueled by sheep manure because wood was scarce. Sources for clay were restricted to the women of the tribe, because pottery was seen as a woman's craft. Traditional methods, forms, and designs were passed down among the women from mother to daughter.

THE MEANING OF MAKING

Dissanayake (1995) suggests that there is an inherent pleasure in making, in using "one's own agency, dexterity, feelings, and judgment to mold, form, touch, hold, and craft physical materials ..." (p. 41). She describes the key abilities and skills progressing developmentally that combine to facilitate man and woman as homo faber. It is through this ability that man and woman use tools both functionally and to leave a mark on the world—an expression of our ideas and our individuality. But the pleasure goes beyond the final product, the craft. It extends to the kinesthetic and sensual involvement with the materials themselves. It offers an alternative to the propensity of the modern world to over-intellectualize and over-analyze human reality.

REFERENCES

Achen, S. T. (1978). *Symbols around us*. New York: Van Nostrand Reinhold Company.

Atkins, J. M. (1994). *Shared threads: Quilting together-past and present*. New York: Penguin Group.

Avedon, E. (1971). *Therapeutic recreation service: An applied behavioral science approach*. Englewood Cliffs, NJ: Prentice-Hall, Inc.

Dissanayake, E. (1995). The pleasure and meaning of making. *American Craft, 55,* 40-46.

Drake, M. (1992). *Crafts in therapy and rehabilitation*. Thorofare, NJ: SLACK, Incorporated.

Halper, V. (1991). The language of containment. In: V. Halper & E. Rossbach (Eds.). *John McQueen: The language of containment* (pp. 41-49). Washington, DC: Smithsonian Institution.

Lindsey, J. L. (1994a). Furman Humphrey and the African American tradition of woodcarving. In: *Works in Progress: Newsletter of the Philadelphia Folklore Project, 1987-1994*. Philadelphia: Philadelphia Folklore Project. (ERIC Document Reproduction Service No. ED 395 872).

Lindsey, J. L. (1994b). Pennsylvania German folk arts: Dowry, quilts and marriage gifts. In *Works in Progress: Newsletter of the Philadelphia Folklore Project, 1987-1994*. Philadelphia: Philadelphia Folklore Project. (ERIC Document Reproduction Service No. ED 395 872).

Rossbach, E. (1986). *The nature of basketry*. West Chester, PA: Schiffer Publishing Std.

Rossbach, E. (1991). Containment and being contained. In: V. Halper & E. Rossbach (Eds.). *John McQueen: The language of containment* (pp. 13-24). Washington, DC: Smithsonian Institution.

Schuman, J. M. (1981). *Art from many hands: Multicultural art projects for home and school*. Englewood Cliffs, NJ: Prentice-Hall, Inc.

Shaw, R. (1993). *America's tradition crafts*. Hong Kong: Hugh Lauter-Levin Associates.

Sorensen, J. (1992). Treating with activity: Tapping your patients' creative muse. *ADVANCE for Occupational Therapists, 8*(32).

Tillman, A. (1973). *The program book for recreation professionals*. Palo Alto, CA: National Press Books.

Messages of Self-Care

Beth P. Velde

Self-care has been described by numerous authors. A consistent theme in these descriptions is that self-care encompasses all those actions that a person does to maintain and sustain health and to offset the impact of disability or disease (Orem, 1991). Those actions take place within the context of a human and physical environment (Fidler, 1994). Therefore, a person's self-care behaviors are inextricably linked with this environment in a pattern of rituals and routines that support the individual's personal lifestyle.

ACTIONS OF SELF-CARE

Discussions of self-care include lists of actions that individuals perform on a daily basis. These include both essential occupations of daily living and functional occupations of daily living. The American Occupational Therapy Association lists tasks that encompass basic self-care behaviors, including grooming, oral hygiene, bathing/showering, toilet hygiene, personal device care, dressing, feeding and eating, medication routine, and sexual expression. Acknowledging the interaction of the individual with his or her human and nonhuman environment, socialization, functional communication, and functional mobility are also included.

Lawton (1971) proposed dividing self-care tasks into two levels, with a second level of functional tasks taking into account the self-care occupations necessary to live in the community. These instrumental occupations of self-care included more complex behaviors, such as use of the telephone, food preparation, housekeeping, laundry, shopping, money management, use of transportation, and medication management.

Fidler has grouped activities regarding the care and maintenance of self into five areas: grooming and dress, management of living space, food and eating patterns, money management, and health management. These are the groupings that will be used in the discussion of the signs and symbols associated with the language of self-care explored in this chapter.

Christiansen (1994), in his discussion of the occupations that make up self-care, emphasizes the importance of the interactions between an individual and his or her human and nonhuman environment as it relates to both the development of a self-identity and the performance of human roles. Self-care is the embodiment of self-identity. The manner in which a person chooses to portray himself or herself to others through dress, hairstyle, jewelry, home decoration, or home management allows the individual to physically and psychologically present his or her identity to others. In a recursive manner, the reaction of others to this presentation helps to shape and reshape the individual's identity. This appears to continue across the lifespan.

GROOMING AND DRESS

Messages regarding self-identity are carried through the objects worn upon the person and objects contained within his or her environment. For example, one's choice of clothing can signal membership in a group. This choice of clothing is seen and understood by others who, in turn, react to it. The reaction varies from understanding and acceptance of the individual as "like me" to a perceived threat. This person is so "unlike me" as to be feared. Recent examples of this have dominated the print news media as school districts attempt to control the dress of students to minimize the effect of gang affiliations and reduce physical aggression while at school. This interpretation of the symbols of dress by the culture has resulted in legislation and adoption of dress codes (Gluckman, 1996).

Some types of popular dress have their origin in the sports arena. In-line skaters and skate boarders began wearing baggy pants and shorts in order to facilitate movement when they skated. Often, these had holes in them from falling or because they were old. Skaters frequently use their skates and boards as transportation, so cargo pants and pants with lots of pockets were advantageous to carry items. In the same manner, putting one's wallet on a chain kept it from falling out while skating. It wasn't long before this type of dress became fashionable outside of skating. Among skaters, those who dress in this manner are grouped in two ways—the authentic skater and the "poser." The poser is a "wanna be," an individual who seeks affiliation with the culture of skating through the symbolism of dress.

Likewise, Csikszentmihalyi and Rochberg-Halton (1981) describe the power of personal symbols in the transformation of feelings that an individual may have about self. Individuals may own objects that they perceive as possessing status. The objects may be endowed through three conditions—the object may be rare, expensive, or it may gain the attention of other people who already have status. Personal objects, such as adornments, include jewelry, fur coats, and designer clothing. Often, an object, such as a piece of antique jewelry, may be one-of-a-kind and, therefore, rare. Because of this, the dollar value of the item is higher than other pieces of jewelry. It is recognized as a sign of status by others who also possess similar items. This may create a special type of consideration, respect, or attention by others. In addition, others may envy the person who possesses the rare item. As a result, the individual may perceive himself or herself in a different manner.

Part of being in the world is relating to and interacting with objects. The objects of adolescence often are those that speak to the development of an identity. Over a 2-month period, Eicher, Barzeriman, and Michelman (1991) interviewed teachers and observed and conducted interviews with 11 high school students in a suburban high school. Through the use of body adornment such as tattoos, objects such as jewelry, and choice of clothing, adolescents experienced others and their social group as being distinct and unique. Some of the categories around which students organized their social groups included jocks, freaks, preppies, nerds, and punks. These groups were identified through the style of clothing, the fabric of the clothing, the choice and placement of bodily adornment, hair style and length, make-up, shoes, and the brand name of clothing.

Two major themes were identified in this research: a hierarchical aspect of adolescent dress and the belief of the adolescents that fluctuation and change regarding the category to which one belonged was possible. The research noted that changes seemed to occur as adolescents approached the end of high school when less attention appeared to be paid to the relationship of dress and social identity. According to the authors, the use of dress by adolescents focused more on the *public self* than on either the *secret self* or *private self.*

Adults and older adults also use dress and bodily adornment to convey a sense of self-identity. Choice of perfume or cologne conveys messages of sensuality, power, and desirability. The role of odor in sexual attraction is well known, and advertisements for colognes and after-shaves play on this, implying their product has aphrodisiac qualities.

The expression of one's sexuality is further accomplished through the signs and symbols of dress and bodily adornment. For men, the location of an earring may signify sexual preference to others and symbolize his feelings of acceptance of his sexual preferences. For women, wearing clothing such as short skirts, halter tops, fishnet stockings, or see-through fabrics may be a sign to others that she is a sexual being and a symbol of her acceptance of her sexuality as a predominant part of her being.

There exists an interesting contrast between attire and personal adornment between other animals and humans. In the human species, the female is frequently the one who is more brilliantly attired, wearing spike heels, short skirts, bright colors, and jeweled nails. All of this to attract another. Among other animals, it is the male who carries the more obvious markings. The drabber appearance of the female allows her to attract less attention, serving to protect the young from predators.

The tie has also carried messages about the man who wears it. Earlier in this century, the bow tie was popular and was considered to be appropriate for both business and formal wear. Currently, the bow tie has fallen from favor for everyday attire. Often, the man who wears it is seen as effeminate, linking the bow with feminine qualities.

In contrast, wearing several layers of sweaters and pants may indicate to others that the person has a need to protect himself or herself from others or that he or she does not have any other place to carry personal possessions. Carrying bundles of clothing, pushing a shopping cart laden with personal possessions, or exhibiting poor hygiene are stigma signals to others who come into contact with the individual. Likewise, the torn seam on a pair of pants represents disorder to the individual wearing them or a lack of concern/pride about one's identity.

The style, color, and pattern of clothing also carry meaning. The older woman currently living in the nursing home frequently is forced to wear a dress that is easy to put on to accommodate for staff time and decreased independence in dressing. Unfortunately, such dresses tend to have a look of uniformity and lack of design, which also are stigma symbols. These may convey to the woman that she is no longer pretty, desirable, or attractive, that her body has become objectified and simply needs to be covered for social acceptability.

Beauty has also become objectified. Numerous books on beauty, dieting, hairstyle, fashion, and make-up represent this country's preoccupation with the beauty myth. Yet, nowhere is the myth of beauty more symbolic than on the reliance of individuals to judge another by his or her face. The face becomes the person, serving as a symbol of who he or she is. Yet, one's own face is always observed through a reflection—in a mirror, a photograph, or through a description of another. The word face serves as a metaphor—"on the face of it," "putting the best face on," "saving face," or "face to face."

Consequently, activities surrounding adorning the face and head acquire special significance. The prevalence of cosmetic surgery is increasing. For women, wearing make-up differentiates both role and choice of activity. More make-up may be worn for work or special occasions, symbolizing to both the self and others that here is a woman in control of her body, of herself. Many women refuse to be seen by others until they have "put on their face." Among men, the taboo of balding continues to receive attention. A balding head represents aging or ill health. Consequently, wigs, hairpieces, and commercial products to grow hair become important aspects of men's grooming rituals.

MANAGEMENT OF LIVING SPACE

An aspect of functional self-care activities is the care and maintenance of one's personal space. This may include a person's bedroom, house, dormitory, or trailer. One example of the power of the symbolism of a bedroom exists in the bedroom of the adolescent. Here is a place where the adolescent maintains a sense of privacy and continues the task of differentiating self from others, particularly the family. Becker (1992) likens the room to a nest where the teen surrounds himself or herself with objects and projects that assist in the discovery process. Bachelard (cited in Becker, 1992) suggests that the room of the adolescent provides a sense of privacy where daydreaming and a construction of self from the inside out begins. This construction of the secret self is an important part of surviving the transition of self. As Becker (1992) describes it,

> *The adolescent's room is a second skin that holds a becoming self, a self in transition. This is a self between selves, one that cannot be grasped because, as yet, it has no visible substance. It is first obvious in what it is not, in what it is leaving behind.* (p. 74)

The maintenance of this private space speaks loudly about its occupant. The choice of objects on the wall may describe an athlete, an artist, or a lover of "Ska" music. The furnishings may symbolize the spirit of the adolescent. A large "boom box" that predominates the room demonstrates the interest of the occupant in auditory entertainment or in drowning out the domestic sounds of others in the household. The earphones hanging on its side provide a way for the adolescent to escape. Like generations of adolescents before him or her, he or she creates symbolic boundaries between self and the world of adults. In music, the lyrics and rhythms are only understood by others in this age group and speak of the dreams, values, and feelings that are yet to be realized. The presence of pictures and significant others links the adolescent to a larger community and symbolizes his or her belonging. The maintenance of the physical space frequently expresses the chaos and disorder of this development period with clothes strewn on the floor and overflowing the drawers. In contrast, the room may be neatly kept with objects and clothing in appropriate places—symbolizing control, at least over his or her immediate environment.

To effectively make the transition from adolescence to adulthood, a separation must occur between the self as perceived as being a child to the self as living in a world where choices are less limited by the parents' wishes. For many adolescents, this comes in conjunction with the physical experience of leaving home and acquiring a physical environment that they can manage and decorate in a style that expresses their identity.

According to Becker (1992), these are both real experiences and symbolic of the phenomenon of transition. The physical act of leaving symbolizes the courage to grow up and to change the parent-child relationship to one that is more equal. The acquisition of this first environment away from the parental home may involve an apartment, a room in a college residence, or the purchase of a house. Later in life, the older adult experiences a different transition. Now, he or she must give up the adult home with all of its symbols of autonomy, family, and self-responsibility to move into a more sheltered environment. The very symbols of transition to adulthood that were valued in adolescence may be losses as the older adult moves into a smaller apartment, condominium, child's residence, personal care home, or nursing home. There may be limited room for personally meaningful objects, and these must be disposed of. This transition may symbolize to the older adult (and to society) that this person is no longer capable of caring for self—a return to the developmental stage of childhood.

The *experience of absence,* whether it is from a parent, spouse, or community results from this change in physical environment. Grieving and a sense of loss may accompany this experience of being absent from home. Perhaps it serves as a vehicle to anticipate and to symbolize the ultimate change—one's own death.

Caring for the home includes cleaning the house, washing the dishes and doing laundry. These tasks have frequently been associated with gender roles. In much of North American society, the woman has cared for the interior of the home. For many women, a clean and tidy house is a symbol that she is meeting the expectations of society. Lucille deView (1996) provides a humorous description of the panic created within a woman when her mother or mother-in-law visits:

> *One minute I was the strong, independent woman bossing people in my job and at home. The next, I was a quivering mess rushing to hide the dirty laundry, scrub the toilet, carry out the trash before my mother strolled up the walk.* (p. 2C)

In the 1940s, women were admonished to "have all your tasks finished before he walks in the door and greet him warmly. Have dinner ready so he can think about it all day long in anticipation. Clear away the clutter" (Bombeck, 1995). Many would suggest that the roles are more equal now, especially with more women in the workforce. Time-based surveys do not support a large change. It is still the woman's role to care for the interior of the home and prepare the meals. As Bombeck further states,

I saw an article in a women's magazine a few weeks ago advising the women of the 90s on how to have a successful marriage. I quote: "Create an atmosphere at home that is both pleasing and comforting. Plan special meals by candlelight and feed the children first. If you know you will be working late, make a pasta salad in the morning that is easy to serve with a warm bread and dessert. Your husband may not always be able to watch his diet. There are special cookbooks you can use to cut his fat intake and keep him healthy." (p. B3)

In contrast, men spend more of their time on the activities of household repairs and yard work. These are more traditionally associated with men's roles and are viewed as acceptable ways for men to contribute to the care of the home. One explanation lies in earlier societies in which men were the typical carpenters, plumbers, and farmers. These work-related roles carried into the household, because it was the man who possessed the needed skills. These tasks also required heavy lifting, use of specialized tools, and involved "dirtier" work. When females were seen as the more fragile of the two sexes and the ones associated with child care, men became the more likely candidates to engage in these activities. They became symbolic of the male's contribution to the home environment.

FOOD AND EATING PATTERNS

Food and eating patterns include the planning, acquisition, preparation, and consumption of food. These activities may occur in isolation or as part of a social setting. Food and the activities related to it symbolize nurturance, growth, and life itself. This is first observed in the suckling of the infant. The infant comes to recognize his or her mother first through the smell and touch of her body as she feeds him or her. For infants who are breastfed, the seeking and finding of the nipple brings comfort and symbolizes security. Every parent recognizes the symbol of a healthy baby—he or she has chubby cheeks, arms, and legs, and responds to his or her parents with visually fixing on the parent's face. When others in the environment observe this, they associate it with good parenting.

The transition of the infant to bottle feeding and subsequently to self-feeding is indicative of development and a move toward independence. Achievement of self-feeding is a major transition from infancy to childhood. Likewise, the increasing ability of the child to participate in activities surrounding food preparation is symbolic of his or her move to independence. When an older individual lacks the skill or abilities to feed himself or herself, this may symbolize for both the individual and a caregiver the return to infancy and results in a tendency to infantilize the individual.

Food serves as a symbol of group identity. This may occur at the national level, where hamburgers and apple pie serve to symbolize the United States and fine cheese and wine to represent France. At the regional level, barbecue and grits are associated with the South and corn on the cob with the Midwest. Religions are also symbolized through foods—vegetarianism with Hinduism or fish on Friday with Roman Catholicism.

Many rituals surround aspects of eating and food preparation. Driver (1991) describes rituals as, "a known, richly symbolic pattern of behavior, the emphasis falling less upon the making and more upon the valued pattern and its panoply of associations" (p. 30). Crepeau (1995) describes three types of rituals—social, sacred and secular, and aesthetic. She further explains that these rituals may exist for an individual or for a group of people. Rituals and their symbols help define the individual and frequently identify him or her with a social group. Ritualized behavior in the social domain characteristic of eating and food preparation frequently revolves around family dinners. The rituals may include a set pattern of behavior with temporal aspects. This includes the shopping, preparing the food by particular family members, setting the dinner table, reciting a blessing, the social experience of sharing the meal, and may include a clean-up ritual with prescribed roles for children, women, and men.

Picnics serve as family rituals for many. Eating, playing, and socializing are key characteristics of the event. Frequently held at familial homes or regional parks, they involve travel by most participants. Often, the trip there is part of the ritual with car games, such as spotting games or license plate bingo. Upon arrival, participants get reacquainted with friends and relatives before engaging in customary games, such as whiffle ball or horseshoes. Typically, men gather together around a game of cards, such as pinochle or poker, or a yard game, such as bocci. Women set up the food, which may include hotdogs and hamburgers from the grill, potato salad, and watermelon. Most often, what is remembered are "the pleasures of gathering with family and friends" (DiBartolomeo, 1995, p. A23).

Food is also involved in sacred/secular rituals. Holy communion with the symbolism of the bread and wine, wedding celebrations with the traditional wedding cake, and funeral wakes with the requisite pot-luck gifts of friends and neighbors are all examples of the relationship of sacred/secular rituals and food.

The Jewish seder is a well-known example of these concepts. Set on the 15th day of the Hebrew month of Nissan, it recalls the momentous meal eaten by the fleeing families of slaves just before their exodus from Egypt. The ritual consists of symbolic food including bitter herbs (maror), vegetables (karpas), bitter vegetables (chazeret), haroset (a mixture of apple, spices, nuts, and wine), shank bone (zeroa), and egg (beitzah). Each of the foods has meaning for the participants. For example, the shank bone represents the sacrifice made in the temple, the haroset is the mortar the slaves were forced to use to construct buildings, and the bitter herbs and vegetables represent the bitterness of the life of slavery. Along with these foods, salt water is placed on the table and is used along with certain foods. This symbolizes the tears of the Israelites during slavery. Four glasses of wine are consumed, one for each of the blessings. Participants are seated with a cushion to the left so they might lean during the seder, imitating free men and nobility.

Hindus also see food consumption as symbolic. Vegetarianism, known in Sanskrit as shakahara, is a practice of both environmental health and ethics. For Hindus, each life form possesses consciousness and energy. To consume meat suggests, "he will eat me in the other world whose flesh I eat here." Vegetarianism is seen as a way to survive with the least injury to other beings.

Cha-no-yu, or the Japanese tea ceremony, is a celebration of the routines of everyday life. This includes making the fire, boiling the tea water, and making and drinking the tea. The tea service is typically austere, representing the simplified beauty of everyday life. In North America, coffee drinking has assumed similar characteristics. Both are gentle acts, acts of simplicity. Drinking coffee or tea is frequently done slowly without gulping. This reinforces a belief that life is best understood when kept to a single moment, a single point in time. Like coffee or tea, life is savored.

Body size and food consumption are closely tied and carry many symbolic connotations. In Western culture, the obese adult is frequently perceived as being lazy, slovenly, and unhealthy. The extremely thin young woman is viewed alternatively as have a psychiatric disorder or being fashion model thin. Beauty is frequently related to body shape, though the symbolism is both culturally, age, and historically related.

As part of the physiological processes tied to feeding and eating, toileting is an issue that also carries symbolic meaning. Manhood and standing to urinate are tied together in Western culture. It is a rite of passage when the young boy is able to join his father at the urinal! Independence in toileting ability is related to a person's view of personal competence and independence.

For women, toileting is frequently a hidden activity. Completed quickly and quietly, it is as if the expulsion of body waste products is embarrassing or somehow soils the participant. Women are known to run the water or crumple paper when using the toilet, a way to cover any sounds associated with the action. Perhaps these attempts to cover the acts relates to society's beliefs that a woman should be seen as clean and pure.

Money Management

In Western culture, money has come to represent success. Everywhere you go, there is money—automatic teller machines (ATMs), banks, and signs for credit cards. Many adults are obsessed with it. Older adults, having spent their youths fixated on not having it, spend endless periods of time worrying about whether they have enough. For them, money means survival. The amount of money charged for a service or earned in a job is equated with a person's value. If too little is charged for a service, someone is likely to reply that "you don't think much of yourself."

The management of money includes several activities, such as check writing, accounting, and budgeting. Being able to write checks to cover expenses is a sign of independence. Balancing one's checkbook signals success. Having enough money left in one's account signals control over the chanciness of economic existence. When someone is without work and money, others see it as a problem, a symbol of weakness and lack of control of one's life. Money can also be seen as a way to show someone else you love him or her or care for him or her.

Purchasing items is tied to money management. To make sure there is enough money on hand to pay for the shopping bills, individuals frequently use a planning process, a budget. This a way to maintain control over one's economic lifestyle. It requires the participant to be aware of the costs of items, project items required, and understand the amount of income and revenue produced. For those individuals less inclined to risk, budgeting is strictly adhered to. Larger items are planned for, and perhaps a small amount is set aside each week or month to limit the amount of loans required. This also requires the ability to delay gratification.

Others spend money as they get it. They are willing to deal with the risk of having no money. In Western culture, the credit card has created another type of shopper. This shopper is able to buy things without the actual exchange of currency. The risk is delayed because the credit card company makes the original purchase in the shopper's name. Beyond signing one's name, it requires little money management skills.

Some types of money appear to have retained their symbolism. Gold as a valued metal is frequently used instead of money. It is the reserve upon which the paper money of the United States was originally based. Azevedo (1998) explains,

> I suggest to friends that they buy an ounce of gold to hold in their hand for a long time. Images will come to the mind. Vacations, things to buy, investments to make. A sense of security. The fear of loss. It's all there in what that one ounce of gold represents, not the gold itself. (p. 2)

HEALTH MANAGEMENT

Health often becomes a topic of interest only in its absence. Concepts regarding health appear to be greatly affected by one's country, culture, economic status, social class, and gender. Too frequently, Western definitions of health see it as an absence of disease. Those in the working class tend to emphasize the functional aspects, such as being able to get necessary tasks done. Those in the middle class tend to stress the psychological aspects and a sense of well-being. Based on survey data from France, laypeople's beliefs in the causation of health lie in a dual explanation involving the external factors of the environmental conditions and germs. In a similar United States study, respondents explained health as a product of a self-determined lifestyle, where release or freedom from stress was an essential component (Rootman & Raeburn, 1994).

Ardell (1996) suggests that health management results in wellness. This is described as an important aspect of self-care and includes aspects such as medication management, exercise, sleep management, and adequate nutrition. Devine (cited in Becker, 1992) studied the exercise experience of young adult women. Based upon interviews and observation, Devine describes three themes around the exercise experience: the dilettante, the social athlete, and the serious athlete.

The *dilettante* is enthralled with the external components of exercise—the clothes, shoes, and equipment. She appears to train and be athletic but does not have the focus to achieve the mind-body experience of a "serious athlete." The objects of exercise serve as signs to others of her athletic interests and may be symbolic of health, belonging, or her worth as a potential mate. Unlike the serious athlete, she does not see exercise as a way of extending herself, of reaching new levels of the mind-body experience.

The *social athlete* participates to be with others. She is there to exercise her body, but not at the expense of the opportunity to socialize. She is most likely to be a part of the group exercise experience. The social athlete perceives exercise as symbolic of her likeness to others whom she values for their healthy lifestyle. She becomes part of the group because of her shared athletic experience.

The *serious athlete* trains to reach both immediate and distant goals. She understands the mind-body connection and works on it. She uses training to identify and overcome both internal and external obstacles. Symbolically, she relates this experience to the integration of all parts of herself—to the achievement of a state of high-level wellness.

Mayo (1992) studied physical activity and African American working women. One of her findings indicated that rehearsal and experimentation with physical activity was an important factor in determining what role exercise would play in their lifestyle. A second factor that impacted the inclusion of physical activity was the "commitment to their exercise partners .... Having someone waiting for them influenced their sense of obligation. Women perceived that time passes faster and activity was more enjoyable when being with other women" (p. 329). Those women in the study who were active developed a process for managing physical activity that included appraising capacity, rehearsing, routinizing, and stabilizing. According to those women who became active after a sedentary childhood, acquiring knowledge, motivation, and resources were important in making lifestyle changes. The women who were active or became active viewed the physical activity as a symbol for increased competence and control over their life experience—for evidence of their increased efficacy.

In contrast, activities that may be perceived as detractors from health are often used to cope with stress or result from the role of caregiver to a family member. These include increased smoking (Cohen, Schwartz, Bromet, & Parkinson, 1991), increased alcohol consumption (Finney & Moos, 1984), substance abuse (Brown, 1989), increased fat/calorie intake (McCann, Warnick, & Knopp, 1990), decreased exercise (Gallant & Connell, 1997), and decreased sleep (Connell, 1994).

Medication management involves activities such as development of a medication routine, establishment of regular medication follow-up by a health care professional, and acquisition of appropriate inoculations against disease. For many, this means the development of a weekly and daily schedule. Some find the characteristic structure of such a routine limiting and see it as a loss of freedom. Others find that the schedule liberates them from worry and allows them time to plan other activities.

Sleep is an essential part of health management. Sleep itself is viewed symbolically as related to death. Individuals who sleep more frequently than others are perceived as lazy or sick. Many would argue that sleeping does not qualify as a true activity. They see it as obligatory and the meeting of a biological need. However, the deprivation of sleep can result in significant health problems. Understanding the activity-based implications of sleep can assist in offsetting potentially functional problems. Managing one's time through the establishment of a regular routine, constructing an appropriate environment for sleep, and creating a daily pattern of activity that is congruent with sleep needs are all types of activities that surround sleep.

OCCUPATIONS OF SELF-CARE AND SELF-MAINTENANCE

The occupations discussed above included grooming and dress, management of living space, food and eating patterns, money management, and health management. To better understand their meaning in your life, an exercise follows. Because self-care and self-maintenance are impacted by age, cultural values, interpersonal relationships, and real/symbolic meaning, it would be useful to complete the questionnaire first for yourself and then interview someone else using the same questions. Compare your responses to his or hers. Where are the similarities and differences? What is your reaction to those? How has self-care and self-maintenance activities impacted the quality of life of each of you?

PERSONAL REPERTOIRE:
THE CARE AND MAINTENANCE OF SELF
by Gail S. Fidler

Respond to the questions listed below. Based upon your responses, evaluate the impact of self-care and self-maintenance tasks on your quality of life and life satisfaction.

Self-Care

1. What percentage (comparative length) of time per day do you spend grooming/dressing?
2. Considering all of the tasks of grooming/dressing, which do you find most enjoyable? Least enjoyable?
3. Do you shower or tub bath? What is the difference? When/under what circumstances do you do each?
4. Do you use a mirror for dressing? Grooming? What types? For what purpose?
5. What factors do you consider when deciding what to wear?
6. How is your "dress" like or different from your peers, parents, others?
7. What is most important to you in relation to dressing/grooming? For whom do you dress/groom?
8. How do you purchase (shop for) your clothing (solo/shared, frequency, planned, spontaneous, type of store)?
9. What about your hair style? What factors influence your choice of style? How is your style like or different from your peers and others? How important is that to you?
10. What cosmetics, cologne, or after-shave do you use? When? Why?

Management of Living Space

1. What furnishings are important to you? Why?
2. Which features are most important to you: color, style, comfort, utility, other?
3. How are your furnishings like or different from your peers, parents, and others?
4. What household tasks and chores do you perform regularly? Why?
5. What tasks do you enjoy? Dislike? Seldom do? Avoid?
6. How would you describe your housekeeping style: neat, tidy, casual, untidy?
7. How were housekeeping tasks managed by your parent(s)? Who was responsible for which tasks? Were you and your siblings involved?
8. Do you share living space with another? If so, how are your housekeeping styles alike? Different? How do these affect your relationship? How do you share/divide tasks?

Food and Eating Patterns

1. To what extent do you engage in meal planning? Cooking? Describe.
2. Do you prepare your own food? Eat out? Rely on another?

continued on Page 120

3. Do you share cooking, meal planning, eating with another/others? Describe.

4. What are your favorite foods? Describe. How did this develop?

5. Do you shop for food? What is that experience like for you?

6. Are there tasks related to obtaining, planning, and eating food that you find enjoyable? Describe. Are there some you find a chore or not enjoyable? Describe.

7. Who did the cooking, shopping, and related tasks in your family?

Money Management

1. Do you manage your own finances? To what extent?

2. What is your characteristic style? Do you plan and adhere to a budget, use credit cards, pay as you go?

3. How do you set spending priorities?

4. What do you do when money runs short? Borrow? From where? Ask for help? From whom? Use credit cards? Live frugally? Which is most characteristic?

5. How is this like or different from when you lived with your parents?

6. How have you managed large purchases, such as a car, your education, a house?

Health Management

1. How much attention do you pay to your health?

2. What do you do regularly to promote your health?

3. Do you exercise? How often? In what ways?

4. Do you have health insurance? How is this financed?

5. Do you consider yourself to be a more active or sedentary person?

6. How health conscious have your parents been?

REFERENCES

Ardell, D. B. (1996). *The book of wellness: A secular approach to spirituality, meaning and purpose*. Amherst, NY: Prometheus Books.

Azevedo, A. (1998, July 20). With what do you buy your money? http://www.goldwarp.com/paradox/buymoney.html.

Becker, C. (1992). *Living and relating: An introduction to phenomenology*. Newbury Park, CA: Sage Publications.

Bombeck, E. (1995, May 1). Are we still supposed to keep his dinner warm? *The Times Leader*.

Brown, S. A. (1989). Life events of adolescence in relation to personal and parental substance abuse. *American Journal of Psychiatry, 146*, 484-489.

Christiansen, C. (1994). A social framework for understanding self-care intervention. In: C. Christiansen (Ed.). *Ways of living: Self-care strategies for special needs* (pp. 1-26). Bethesda, MD: American Occupational Therapy Association.

Cohen, S., Schwartz, J. E., Bromet, E. J., & Parkinson, D. K. (1991). Mental health, stress, and poor health behaviors in two community samples. *Preventive Medicine, 20*, 306-315.

Connell, C. M (1994). Impact of spouse care giving on health behaviors and physical and mental health status. *The American Journal of Alzheimer's Care and Related Disorders & Research, 9*, 26-36.

Crepeau, E. B. (1995). Rituals (Module 6). In: C. B. Royeen, *The Practice of the future: Putting occupation back into therapy*. Bethesda, MD: American Occupational Therapy Association.

Csikszentmihalyi, M., & Rochberg-Halton, E. (1981). *The meaning of things: Domestic symbols and the self*. New York: Cambridge University Press.

de View, L. S. (1996, March 5). When moms visit, daughters go into cleaning frenzy. *The Times Leader*.

DiBartolomeo, A. (1995, August 3). It's not the food or the sun that make cookouts fun. *Philadelphia Inquirer*.

Driver, T. F. (1991). *The magic of ritual*. San Francisco, CA: Harper.

Eicher, J., Barzeriman, W., & Michelman, J. D. (1991). Adolescent dress part II: A qualitative study of suburban high school students. *Adolescence, 26*, 103.

Fidler, G. S. (1994). Preface. In: C. Christiansen (Ed.). *Ways of living: Self-care strategies for special needs* (pp. v-vi). Bethesda, MD: American Occupational Therapy Association.

Finney, J. W., & Moos, R. H. (1984). Life stressors and problem drinking among older adults. In M. Galanter (Ed.). *Recent developments in alcoholism* (Vol. 2, pp. 267-288). New York: Plenum.

Gallant, M. P., & Connell, C. M.(1997). Predictors of decreased self-care among spouse care givers. *Journal of Aging & Health, 9*, 373-396.

Gluckman, I. B. (1996). *Dress codes and gang activity. A legal memorandum*. Reston, VA: National Association of Secondary School Principals. (ERIC Document Reproduction Services No. ED 393199).

Lawton, M. P. (1971). The functional assessment of elderly people. *Journal of the American Geriatrics Society, 19*, 465-481.

Mayo, K. (1992). Physical activity practices among American black working women. *Qualitative Health Research, 2*, 318-333.

McCann, B. S., Warnick, R., & Knopp, R. H. (1990). Changes in plasma lipids and dietary intake accompanying shifts in perceived workload and stress. *Psychosomatic Medicine, 52*, 97-108.

Orem, D. E. (1991). *Nursing: Concepts of practice*. New York: McGraw-Hill.

Rootman, I., & Raeburn, J. (1994). The concept of health. In: A. Pederson, M. O'Neill, & I. Rootman (Eds.), *Health promotion in Canada: Provincial, national & international perspectives* (pp. 56-71). Toronto, Canada: W. B. Saunders Press.

ADDITIONAL READING

Brown, L. (1994). *Meeting at the crossroads*. Cambridge, MA: Harvard University Press.

Frank, G. (199). The personal meaning of self-care. In: C. Christiansen (Ed.). *Ways of living: Self-care strategies for special needs* (pp. 27-49). Bethesda, MD: American Occupational Therapy Association.

Rookus, M. A., Burema, J., & Frijters, J. E. (1988). Changes in body mass index in young adults in relation to number of life events experienced. *International Journal of Obesity, 12*.

CHAPTER 10

Voices of the Arts

Gail S. Fidler

Any attempt to explore some of the meaning and messages inherent in the arts is at once a complex and challenging undertaking. The intrigue of the arts is ageless; and, thus, there is an impressive abundance of information stretching from the beginning of time to this day. Furthermore, it is important, especially for our purpose, to differentiate the individual arts while retaining their relatedness and their meaning as a whole. Peloquin (1996) expresses this when she writes, "Listening to a symphony is an act that is different from reading a novel or contemplating a sketch. Yet the likeness among these acts—that each is art—make the world of art" (p. 656).

A sampling of the literature concerning the arts reveals a marked agreement among scholars regarding their significant role in the development of human capacity. Hayman (1969), in the remarkable volume *The Arts and Man*, provides an excellent overview of the value of the arts in the life of the individual and in the formation and recording of cultures. This writer has identified a number of factors as hallmarks of engagement with the arts. As this chapter unfolds, it will become evident that, although there may be different semantics, there is a consensus that attests to these processes as inherent in defining the meaning and role of the arts. The following descriptions have been adapted from Hayman's (1969) original material.

- *Discovery*—Art increases one's sensitivity and awareness. It is a means of clarifying and refining ideas. For example, in producing a crayoning, a painting, a song, or an object of clay either as a child, a novice adult, or artist, the act reflects what the performer has discovered about his or her world and about himself or herself. Canaday (1964) views art as a history of self-discovery, involving experiences of learning to see, to explore, to compare, and to contrast—the pencil, the brush, the hand, and the body are all explorers.

- *Intensification*—Involvement within the arts intensifies and sharpens our senses (Hjort and Laver, 1997). As we listen to a Mozart composition, create a watercolor, watch a Kirov performance, or sing in a chorus, our senses are heightened, and both emotional and intellectual responses are triggered.

- *Expression*—Art is a voice of self and a voice of a culture (Highwater, 1978; Hayman, 1969). Individual abilities, points of view, and preferences distinguish the individual as well as the culture. The theme of art represents and affirms individual uniqueness and cultural unity, and its message thus gains universal acceptance. Every individual and every culture gives form to feelings, perceptions, and thought through various art forms.

- *Record*—The role of the arts as a recorder of events and of cultural history is readily evident. The cave drawings, paintings, sculptures, music scores, dances, and theatre endure and exist as a record, a profile of time and its events. According to Marquet (1986), what we know of ancient societies, we know because of the artifacts they have left to us.

- *Communication*—Hayman views all forms of art as communication, pointing out that ideas, values, perceptions, and feelings are symbolically expressed and shared with others. Symbolic messages as we have noted go well beyond words. Lomax (1964), Hanna (1987), Sparshott (1997), and Highwater (1978), among others, consider communication to be a major and inherent characteristic of the arts. What endures through the ages are those productions, those art forms of theatre, music, dance, and the visual arts whose symbolic messages find consensus among people.

- *Interpretation*—The great variety of art and art forms presents us with many different visions and perceptions about nature and human experiences. To be made aware of and come to know different interpretations, different ways of perceiving events and conditions, expands our own and society's vision and understanding. Read (1970), in particular, emphasizes that this characteristic of the arts comprises a crucial aspect of the arts as education.

- *Reformation*—Art seeks to change and reform. Hayman explains arts' symbolic process of reformation of change, saying "the artist takes the pigments, the fibers, wood, clay, rock, and metal from their natural states and gives them new form—takes the everyday visions, sounds, and values of man and reforms them as well" (p. 21). Certainly, a mission of the arts, its voices, and its messages is to heighten awareness, expand horizons, and influence and alter how one thinks and feels.

- *Enhancement*—The creation of aesthetic objects and aesthetic experiences and the portrayal of beauty is indeed an objective of artistic endeavor. The sensory and intellectual challenge to judge what is beautiful unites individuals in agreement and, at the same time, clarifies individuality in seeing things in a different way. Peloquin (1996) articulates this process as coming to view self and one's work with new eyes.

- *Order*—The arts give order and coherence to things and events. And, order and structure are essential to the creation of any art form. The rhythm that molds movement into dance, the structure and time that transforms sound into music, and the juxtaposition of color, line, and form are the essential orderliness of art; and, in turn, the aesthetic experiences enable the human being to bring parts of life and thought together in an ordered structure (Lomax, 1968; Hayman, 1969).

- *Integration*—Integrating the orderly parts into a whole is essential in the arts and in our daily living. "The synthesis of emotion and intellect, establishing relationships among fantasy, thought, and imagination, and the physical world of objective reality is both a process and function of art" (Hayman, 1969, p. 25). These processes are essential in both creating art and ensuring its communicative power (Arieti, 1976).

Peloquin (1996) has argued that engagement in art is integral to the development of empathy. This thesis finds support, Peloquin contends, in the very nature of the art experience. Art evokes many sensory and affective responses. It affords a connection with the feelings of others and with one's own inner processes, making it possible to see self and one's world with new eyes. Art reflects and builds a common understanding and, at the same time, affirms the idiosyncratic nature of a human experience, thus enabling appreciation of differences.

The use of metaphor in art is understood as a means of stimulating and stretching imagination, which, in turn, generates new and fresh connections and enhances the capacity to understand. As in literary fiction, the call of art to enter the virtual world of the artist offers experiences of observing, reflecting on, and being engaged with many aspects of life. Peloquin (1996) concludes that the literature confirms three fundamental rules of art: reliance on bodily senses, the use of metaphor, and experience with virtual worlds. The relevance of these conjectures to the 10 characteristics of art previously described is clearly evident.

VOICES OF THE ARTS

Art as teacher, as fundamental and integral to education, has been an overriding theme of Herbert Read for many decades. His acclaimed studies have served as resources for numerous scholars of the arts. In one particular publication, Read (1970) states that the inherent value of art is that of teacher, because art in all of its forms engages and develops all human senses and mental processes. As noted in Chapter 1, this scholar has considered the visual and plastic arts as significant in the development and maturation of visual acuity and touch. Music and dance are described as enabling and refining auditory and motor skills, drama as nurturing articulation, and crafts as stimulating and engaging thought processes. Read (1970) emphasizes how the sensory and cognitive learning and development that occurs from experiences in the arts develops and enriches perceptions, imagination, feelings, and thoughts. Furthermore, the action or doing nature of the arts is understood as a force that initiates and supports expression and communication of ideas, values, customs, and sensitive judgments. This calls to mind Moore and Anderson's aesthetic objects category of socializing activities and their view of the aesthetic experiences nurturing the capacity to assess and make valuative judgments.

The meaning and significance of the aesthetic factor, according to Read (1970), are to be found in the fundamental act of apprehending. This act is explained as a process of perceiving, evolving an image, and responding physiologically and meteorically to that image and effectively ordering and organizing these. Thus, the creative activities, such as art, dance, drama, and music, become teacher and catalyst in the development of human capacity. We are reminded that Plato viewed art and society as inseparable, arguing that society depends on art as a binding and fusing force. Read (1970) reiterates this theme when he states that "only in so far as a society is sensitive to the arts do ideas become accessible to it" (p. 62).

It is intriguing to note that in early societies—in pre-Columbian America, Africa, Oceana, even into the middle ages—there was no "art": There were no objects created for the purpose of observation or contemplation. What was created were instrumental objects. Objects as an integral part of living were produced and used for a purpose, such as weapons, cooking utensils, sacred objects used in worship, masks, and ceremonial garments. Only when they were no longer used, when they became cultural artifacts, were they viewed as art. Very few objects were made exclusively to be contemplated as in the tradition today. Only in later societies were objects created solely for the purpose of contemplation and interpretation (Marquet, 1986).

The process of creating and producing in the arts involves several neurological processes, each influenced by idiosyncratic brain function and personal experiences. These have been described by Arieti (1976) as including:

- *Perception*—The faculty of apprehending how one views a scene, an object, or event
- *Imagery*—To hold an image, to store a visual memory of what has been seen
- *Imagination*—To mentally put together parts that were not there originally
- *Affect*—To attach feeling to these
- *Cognition*—The process of structuring and ordering meaning. Read (1970) views feelings as the organizer of these processes, and Arnheim (1969) calls perception visual thinking and defines this dynamic as the coming together of the senses in the process of creating.

Arieti (1976) points out that these interactive processes explain why even the very early representational art style was never photographic. The interrelated processing of sensory, affective, and cognitive phenomena, no matter how concrete or abstract, Arieti asserts, results in a product that inevitably reflects the inner process of the creator. This scholar explains creativity as a synthesis of the irrational, primitive unconscious with the logical, rational, and cognitive mechanisms of the conscious mind. Modern art, he says, exemplifies this fusion. No matter how deeply the artistic endeavor plunges into the primary process, "it rises again to attune to the secondary process. The details merge into a unity, the parts form a whole, and the concrete becomes the incorporation of the abstract" (p. 223). Chagall's paintings are used as an example. They do not represent the ordinary aspects of things, reality is disregarded, and the fantasy, imaginative primary processes, holds sway. However, Arieti reminds us that then the magic of Chagall takes over. "His language while abstruse is actually understood the world over—ancient Jewish values, Russian folklore, and French innovations blend and harmonize—in a spirit of joy that calls forth a universal response" (p. 224). For the student who is seriously interested in the creative processes, this volume is, in itself, a creative challenge.

Creating in the visual and plastic arts is a solitary process, requiring and nurturing the distancing of self from the activity of the immediate here and now reality. This solitary experience encourages the development, refinement, and reliance on inner ideational capacities. To portray a landscape, carve form from stone, or sculpt a figure out of clay requires contemplative solitude (Nadeau, 1993). This requirement identifies quite clearly the single person as architect, as creator of the end product and, thus, heightens the sense of self-agency, ownership, and the ability to make things happen. The visual and plastic arts live and endure because their voices speak with meaning, relevance, and beauty to others. Each production is an individual statement of the artist's inner processes, experiences, and concerns within the context of his or her culture. It is a uniquely personal statement expressed through visual imagery with line and color, forming a mask that is uniquely self (Nadeau, 1993).

By contrast, dance, music, and drama require a sensitive awareness of and connectedness with others in formalized, organized, and sequential patterns. In these art forms, the audience frequently becomes as important as the creator or performer. However, Marquet (1986) reminds us that art is not simply an independent entity created by the artist, but rather a mental construct agreed upon by a group of people. It is not separate from the culture in which it is created any more than its creator is an independent entity. "Reality is the mental construction of a group, the consensus of one's contemporaries, and art is part of a socially constructed reality" (p. 32).

VOICES OF DANCE

Dance, music, and drama require a sensitive awareness of a connectedness with others in formalized, organized, and sequential patterns. In these art forms, the audience frequently becomes as important as the creator or performer. Dance is a characteristically different art form as compared with the visual arts. It is an activity involving sensory awareness, body awareness, and flexibility, a process of getting in touch with one's body. It requires the joining of the body with feelings, thus developing body control and a sense of being in control of self. Through movement, dance tells our story, who we are, our culture, our belonging, our feelings, and thoughts. In dance, the body becomes a vehicle of expression (Warren & Corten, 1993). Movement is a part of all behavior. We are constantly engaged in motions in our everyday living. Lomax (1968) points to the discernable relationship between dance styles and work styles. Warren and Corten (1993) suggest that washing our faces, working in the garden, or baking bread, for instance, can be viewed as our own special dances.

The body is an instrument of expression and a vehicle for discovery. Body movement plays a critical role in our growth and development, in the exploration of the world around us, and in coming to know our capabilities. We are all aware of the link between emotion and body movement. Our gestures, how we stand, and the way we move all express quite eloquently what we are feeling. Warren and Corten (1993) use the term "sub-text" to convey this dynamic of nonverbal communication. Highwater (1978) supports the thesis that action precedes conception, affirming that body movement is the most fundamental and expressive act. The innate physiology of movement and the sensorimotor and proprioceptive input seemed to be the basis for primal people to know movement as magic and for Westerners to know it as a powerful force in human experience. Acknowledging and understanding sub-textual messages is fundamental to understanding dance as a forceful expresser and communicator across all languages and all cultures and as basic to the creation of all dance forms. The study of movement led to Laban's (1956) creation of movement analysis. This system for analyzing movement formed the basis for most choreography and has contributed to a more sophisticated understanding of the use of body movement to convey meaning (Bartenieff, 1980).

Studies of ancient cultures and the history of art forms suggest that, although dance and music are closely related, dance, or at least body movement to convey messages, preceded song and came well before speech (Lomax, 1968). Song is the natural evolution from movement. Movement forces sound and thus song (Highwater, 1978). In less industrialized societies, there is an obvious relationship between dance styles and work styles. Movements that are an integral part of the everyday work of the people are translated and organized into dances. Other movements of everyday life are also structured into dances, such as relating, grooming, sexuality, etc. In more highly organized, complex cultures, the relationship of daily living activities to the dance is more obscure, more symbolically displayed. Lomax (1968) studied the similarity of work and dance styles in 21 different cultures, confirming that the movement style in dance is a crystallization of the most important and crucial pattern of everyday activities. Contained in this study is a most remarkable description of an Eskimo and a Trajdjik dance. Eloquently demonstrated is the relationship of dance and work movements, of how dance movements replicated and symbolically displayed the movements and social patterns of the Eskimo hunter and in contrast the Trajdjik farmer (pp. 226-227).

The Kachina dances are rituals of the American Southwest Indians. They are part of an elaborate religious lifestyle. "The creative power of rituals like the Kachina dances lies in their capacity to awaken imagery within the person, to compound mystery with more mystery, and to illuminate the unknown without reducing it to the common place" (Highwater, 1978, pp. 18, 19). Ritual is a symbolic transformation of experiences.

Dance is composed of those gestures, postures, and movements most characteristic and most essential to all activities and issues of living. All body movement communicates the mores, customs, values, beliefs, and role relationships found in a given culture. The critical shapes and modes of body movement either in an organized dance or in one's own daily movement and posture are culturally determined and learned (Lomax, Bartenieff, & Paulay, 1968; Sparshott, 1997).

The dance in any culture or historical era is always something inseparable from the views of the dancers, their reference groups, and certainly the particular meanings assigned by the pervading culture. Dance is distinctive for the way in which the performer cannot avoid being directly present in the act. Additionally, "every member of an audience brings to a performance every thing that he or she happens to be and every member of the dance group will contribute to the making of the dance—all the perspectives and prejudices that make them what they are" (Sparshott, 1997). The cultural influences on dance form can be examined further by looking at styles of dance from the perspective of movement analysis (Bartenieff, 1980; Laban, 1956). According to these artists and Lomax (1968), the baseline from which dance activity has developed consists of two basic body postures. In one, the body trunk is treated as one unit, a solid, inflexible trunk that provides support for up and down, back and forth movements. Speed, strength, and weight are the primary considerations. The everyday movements of, for example, hunters, fishermen, and stevedores are readily expressed in this form with thrusting, pushing, lifting, hurling, and pounding movements.

What dances today are based on this style? American and European folk dance? The Irish dance? Tap dancing?

The second movement classification, by contrast, includes clear-cut twists at the waist, undulation, upper and lower limb movements, and flexible, fluid body rotations of rhythm. These are the everyday movements of the cattle herders, steer roping, the agricultural work of sowing seed, planting, hoeing, and harvesting.

What dances today seem to be based on this style? The ballet? The waltz? Which dances seem to combine both styles?

Dance experience flows from a culture's earliest perception of itself and the environment from which it was born. The history of dance is linked to a broad range of cultural forces (Highwater, 1978, p. 19). The public television series on dance shown a few years ago was a magnificent showing of dance as a universal language in all of the beauty of its unique history and cultures. The dynamic quality and the power and force of the expressive quality of dance is magnificently articulated by Sommer in her review of *Manhattan Taps'* recent production (1998). The metaphors of the articles' title strikingly communicate the essence of dance. And Sommer's review is a telling description of the codes of meaning inherent in dance. The melody of movement styles so characteristic of much of modern day dance is evident. Sommer contends the works, which blend American and African rhythms, spiced with Afro-Cuban dancing, are described as "a rambunctious hybrid, distinguished by its rhythm which transitions the dancers into percussive musicians whose feet are their instruments." Because this form of dance can absorb all varieties of music and dance movements, "it can remain free and connected to the larger social context"—"dance you can hear, music you can see—rhythm speaks a language that anyone can understand."

What can we say about the dance patterns that are and/or have been popular in the United States? What interpersonal roles, social values, and customs are reflected in, for example, the Charleston, the Jitterbug, the social dancing of the 1950s, the 1980s, and 1990s? What are some of the significant differences among these? What characteristics seem to remain constant?

VOICES OF MUSIC

The origins of all modern dance are all within the idea that all art is the expression of emotion. Dance today is eclectic and multimedia and, of course, related to established systems of meaning and expressions, methods and forms.

As we engage in this analysis, in all probability, the music associated with each style comes to mind. Music and dance most usually go hand in hand, so it seems logical to turn now to a glimpse of music and meaning. Both music and dance are given coherence by two very basic elements, the organizing elements of repetition and rhythm and their sociocultural theme. Dance is viewed as the most redundant, formally organized system of body communication, and song is seen as the most repetitious and formally patterned of all oral communication (Hanna, 1988; Lomax, 1968).

Both music and dance are an integral part of many rituals, such as religious ceremonies, holiday observances, marriages, harvests, births, and deaths, each symbolizing a community consensus. "Through music, the human being worships God, releases exuberance through drinking songs and dance, falls in love to music, marches to war, shares solitude, celebrates in ceremony, and communicates" (Menuhin 1969, p. 167). Song and dance patterns also vary in relation to culture-specific social and interpersonal styles. Songs in particular reflect a difference, for instance, in tonal quality, melody, rhythm, and tempo, depending on the nature of the audience. Music and dances for an all-male group or mixed genders, for royalty, for the higher echelons of the social network, or for the ordinary social group vary accordingly. Similar to dance, there is a definite link between the norms and style of song and the work style of the people. The song, the music, and the dance all reflect the social structure, the hierarchy of a society. The more complex the social-political structure, the more varied is that culture's music and dance. The research of Lomax reveals such variations in style, including the simple repetitive theme and the ballads and stories of more complex, diverse, hierarchical societies. Music both expresses emotion and is the cause or source of emotion. A musical performance is a public, cognitive, performance act into which the audience enters as an interpreter. It is similar to dance, a collective phenomenon. As a cause, music elicits bodily sensory and motor responses. It is, in this sense, an individual experience (Hjort & Lauer, 1997).

Song is usually a statement of a group. It serves as a focal point for organizing a natural response and presenting a consensus. The text songs, those with a message, are limited to those events, issues, concerns, attitudes, and feelings on which the community is in maximum accord (Lomax, 1968). We can name many examples that illustrate this point. The songs of Peter, Paul, and Mary and Joan Baez are all written and sung to reflect the consensus among the youth of the 1960s. As values and attitudes among the mainstream of our society changed, many of these songs became our folk songs. The Negro spirituals reflecting within the sharing community a consensus of deep pathos, a unity of feelings, nostalgia, and intense concerns are a superb example of such transitions. As we began to change our social beliefs and values, the beauty and messages of these songs have taken a special place in our culture.

When a community sings, it seems to make many statements about the level of complexity that strongly affects every aspect of its life. "In performing a song, the person reminds self of the kind of community one comes from and its level of achievement" (Lomax, 1968, p. 163).

Formal orchestral presentation seems to indicate a firmer, more complex, and rigid social structure. Furthermore, according to Lomax, the number of various types of instruments in the largest orchestras reflects the level of social stratification. Thus, for example, the growth of the symphony orchestra in Europe and subsequently in the United States symbolized the rise of a rich and powerful elite and glorification of leader, king, or dictator.

What inferences can be drawn from these observations regarding the sociocultural messages of the music styles that are part of our culture?

- *What comparisons of cultural consensus can be made among, for instance, rock, country, jazz, and classical music?*
- *What is the message of the high-volume, repetitious pulsating beat, vigor, and forcefulness of rock?*
- *What about the ballad, or the soft, swinging, fluid, repetitious melody of country music?*
- *In what ways are these characteristically different from jazz, the music of Wynton Marsalis or Yanni, the creations of Beethoven or Verdi?*

In terms of the performer, instrumental music is different from that of song. Lomax (1968) explains this difference "as song being produced by the body, pouring out from the throat, and shaped by the lips and tongue. In contrast, instrumental music occurs outside of the body, the instruments are 'literally manipulated'" (p. 152).

Does this then imply that there is an experiential and psychological difference between playing a horn that is blown and playing a piano or violin? What are the differences? What are the differences among oneself being the instrument as in singing, blowing a horn, manipulating an instrument such as the piano or violin, or conducting to create the music?

These questions lead to other associations. For instance, we suggest that there is a relationship between a style of music and the instruments associated with that style. The piano, for example, relates to all music, while the violin is most frequently associated with classical and country music. The clarinet is associated with jazz and classical; and the trumpet is associated with band, sacred, and alertive sound. What other relationships can be made? These associations have some influence on the meaning that an instrument has for a given individual.

What examples came to mind?

Another dimension of meaning emerges from consideration of the manner in which the instrument must be managed in order to produce music. We can agree that achieving this end (making music) requires a certain degree of talent and skill that derives from one's brain structure and neurophysiology (Hermann, 1988). An affinity for and interest in a particular instrument can, in all probability, be attributed to this factor as well as one's personal sociocultural experiences. One added consideration in discerning meaning is the distinguishable operational requirements of an instrument such as shaking, blowing, hitting, pounding, and the like. It seems reasonable to conjecture that if body movements and posture have special significance in dance and drama, then the forceful blowing of a trumpet, the beating of a drum, or the stroking of a harp, for instance, would be equally meaningful, especially to the performer.

What conjectures can you offer? What associations can be made related to the violin, the piano, French horn, base drum? Others? What is your favorite musical instrument? What is special about it?

Writing about the contribution of music to humanity, Menuhin (1969) speaks with the eloquence of the true artist and musician. He addresses those elements or characteristics of music that have great significance in reflecting the human condition and shaping humanity. Music is viewed as a process of making order out of chaos, because rhythm imposes unanimity, melody continuity, and harmony compatibility. The relationship of music to life is described by intriguing examples of relationships between musical elements, human physiology, and the fluctuating elements of work and rest. The impact of sound and, thus, the ability of music to penetrate deeply into the mind and profoundly affect emotions is, Menuhin believes, more profound than any other impression. Music is acknowledged as making it possible to know and understand people and worlds unknown to us. This theme is similar to Peloquin's virtual world and to Hayman's description of interpretation. The human urge for self-expression and for sharing such experiences with others is viewed as happening through the improvisation that occurs in spontaneous jazz, improvised instruments, and the exploration of sounds and rhythms. One can note some excellent examples of such exploration and discovery, including the popular stage show *Stomp*, an exhilarating production of sound and rhythm. Menuhin tells us that music as sound occupies us quite literally, physically, and spiritually. Certainly, the irresistible urge of audiences to stand, shout, and stomp in response to this production testifies to the validity of that observation. Carl Orff's creative work in guiding individuals to create song from everyday sounds and rhythm and incorporating music, dance, and mime is a delightful experience in shared improvisation and spontaneity. Menuhin calls attention to the ability of music to reflect every aspect of life, every occurrence, "a child's cry, a peal of thunder, love as in a Schubert song or the intellect of a Bach fugue, adding that, the quality of sound is identical to touch, rendered as warm, cold, silken, velvety, sensuous, or dry" (p. 169).

Finally, this artist addresses the critical and essential value of music and art as the bedrock of education and, thus, in the creation of humanity. In this brief summary, it is not possible to do justice to his material. It should be read and studied as he has written it, in all of its poetic, artistic, and insightful style.

The arts in education have continued to be a topic of concern for many artists and educators. Addressing the diminishing classical music audience, the reality that fewer students are studying music in the United States and Europe, and fewer classical recordings are being sold, Griffiths (1998) suggests that some of the reason is that the music culture has come to value only the traditional. He contends that, for this culturally based reason, exposure to the best new classical music remains inadequate, and that the lack of a new Beethoven is not the cause of music's stagnation but rather a symptom—a symptom of the lack of music education in our schools and, thus, the lack of exposure in the young to music. He makes a strong plea for encouraging and strengthening music education in our schools. He asserts that music teaches the ability to listen and that listening to and performing enables skills related to mathematics and language. Being involved in a performance provides significant learning about presenting oneself in public, how to argue a case, fostering skills of discernment, and how to work with others toward a common goal. The value of music in and of itself is acknowledged as teaching how to express a thought or feeling and phrasing that thought so that it can be understood and shared with others. Griffiths contends that music experiences help one to discover the importance of things that have no physical existence or monetary worth. It is this element that Menuhin calls communicating the intangible.

VOICES OF DRAMA

It is very likely that most of us can remember those special early years when pretend play was so much a part of our world. The drape of a scarf over our head, small feet in a parent's shoe, and voila! The magic transformation to Cinderella, angel, witch, or superman was complete. The make believe of play acting, the transformation of self into the persona of another made it exciting and safe to explore a variety of feelings, behaviors, and ideas and catch a glimpse of one's capacity and potential. The plays, talent shows, and skits produced for parents are testimony to the enduring role of imagination in the testing and exploration of one's inner and outer worlds. These imaginative leaps continue at an increasing level of sophistication, influencing our understanding of self, of social and career roles.

In drama, imaginative thought and play acting become organized action. Warren (1993) describes it as a highly expressive, dramatic display of thoughts, feelings, and beliefs that are managed and controlled by formalized external factors, such as the script, staging directions, the sequencing of time, and the role of others. While drama requires the ability to enter the skin of another, to identify with and take on the character, feelings, and values of author, it also requires being able to differentiate self from the role—to re-emerge from the journey richer for the experience and wiser about self (Warren, 1993). This observation is very similar to the perspective of Arieti that was referenced earlier in this chapter regarding the capacity and necessity of the visual artist to emerge from the primitive sensory immersion.

Drama cannot exist in solitude. It requires more than one individual to be part of the experience as actor or audience. It is an interactive communication process comprising both verbal and nonverbal behaviors to express its message. Like other forms of art, it is sociocultural communication, reflecting those issues, concerns, and interests of the times as well as issuing a clear statement about how these should be expressed and the appropriateness of the telling (Warren, 1993). The style and theme of the play, what is popular and successful, is a barometer of the society in which it is written and produced. There are and have been productions that express a particular fad as theme and are short-lived, a momentary entertainment. However, there are many more dramas that continue to challenge producers, actors, and audiences over the years because of the timelessness of their theme. The ability to artfully portray the dilemmas, feelings, and thoughts that are part of living makes the plays of great artists, such as Shakespeare, Chekov, Shaw, Ibsen, and O'Neill, timeless.

The theatre is a microcosm of life. Its appeal is in its portrayal of the mysteries and intrigues of human life. Melnitz (1969) reminds us that drama and theatre are as old as the world is itself, beginning with the first man who thought that by imitating animals he could increase the availability of game. Drama, similar to the other arts, has grown and become more complex in story and presentation as society has grown more complex and sophisticated. Changes in the form and style of the theatre moved like art, dance, and music from the representational, imitative form to more elaborate abstract presentations. This development is beautifully described in a passage from the writing of Melnitz (1969). As drama moves beyond imitative magic,

> *man discovers how to use dance and music as well as masks in rituals that he hopes will bring rain and increase his crops. He invents initiation ceremonies that require dialogue. His ancestors become gods and he worships them with song and dance. Worship breeds myths, and myths must be acted out—at last he is devising tragedy, and after that Bacchic comedy, and then plays that are acted just for the fun of it.* (p. 123)

The theatre is a multifaceted art form combing the visual arts in stage sets, music, dance and movement, and the art of dialogue. It is, furthermore, a complicated medium because it must constantly renew itself. In our world of today, its success depends on its ability to offer a wide repertoire, reflecting the complexity of our society and its varied and different concerns and interests. It is interesting and encouraging to note that the youth of today have discovered theatre. Acting is seen as a noble, noteworthy career, and applicants to the schools of drama in the United States have more than doubled in the late 1990s.

What sociocultural changes might contribute to this move? Can you relate this interest to aspects of your daily lifestyles?

Further social and cultural change seems to be reflected in the growing popularity of musical comedy presentations given by traveling road companies. *The New York Times* (Schiff, 1998) has reported on this developing trend at length, noting that the performing arts centers in many large cities have changed their traditional scheduling priorities to accommodate the large audiences attending these productions. The significance of such change is marked by the fact that performing arts centers have been built and supported for years by symphony and opera patrons. These classical music companies and their supporters are now having to find less adequate space and facilities.

In concert with such movements are the marked changes in and diminishing number of classical radio stations. Many have converted to all news programs, and the few remaining ones have significantly altered their musical choices to primarily background listening compositions rather than the more musically complex classics (Schiff, 1988).

How might these changes be explained? Are the predictions of Read (1970) and the explanations of Griffiths (1998) adequate explanations?

Film is closely related to the theatre. Many screen stars begin their careers in live theatre, and a significant number of acclaimed plays have been successfully adapted to film. However, the stature of film took decades to develop. It was originally viewed not as an art form, but rather as "pool hall" entertainment according to Kosinsen (1969). The audience demanded fast-moving action, exaggerated events, and slapstick comedy. As filming techniques improved, a wider audience was attracted, and news, travelogues, along with the villain-maiden escapades began to be the principle attraction. It was more like a newspaper than an art and was treated in like manner. However, the increasing sophistication of filming began to bring about a significant change in script as well as in the acting, and film began to be an art rather than simply entertainment. Audiences began to expect that the cinema related more to their lives, and the substance of films continued to increase. Nevertheless, the cinema of today and its television counterpart acknowledge the mass appeal of entertainment, and consequently "high" drama, movement, and speed have a high priority in the industry. The burgeoning of young film directors creating films related to the interest and concerns of today's youth and young adults is testimony to the entertainment power of fast action and its accompanying loud sound.

In drama, the joining of the actor and audience and the identification of the spectator with the actors create a bond, a unity in time and place. Drama demands a sense of community, and the theatre can create an environment so that such integration can occur. This collaborative nature of drama supports the development of a collective togetherness (Warren, 1993). Similarly, we have seen throughout this chapter how music, art, dance, and now drama by the uniqueness of the aesthetic experience, require and enable a togetherness, a sharing, and a sense of community.

ASSIGNMENTS

The following tasks are designed to broaden and enrich students' perceptions and learning.

They provide an opportunity for the learner to reflect on his or her own personal experiences. Order and organize these reflections to achieve some perspective on meaning. Share these with others and gain from the analysis and diversity of thought.

When these assignments are placed at relevant intervals throughout the chapter, they add considerable dimension to the study.

Music: Cultural and Personal Connections

1. Briefly identify your preferred music style (e.g., jazz, rock, classical, country).
2. How did you learn about this music, and how long has it been your favorite?
3. Is your involvement as a performer, listener, or both?
4. Do you listen to and/or perform any other style of music? How frequently and what kind?
5. Briefly describe your preferred style of music, commenting on at least the following characteristics:
   - Sociocultural orientation
   - Volume
   - Rhythm
   - Tempo
   - Melody
   - Interpersonal orientation
   - Lyrics
6. Interview an individual whose music style is different from yours (e.g., an older adult, friend, or relative). Ask this person to describe his or her preferred and frequently used music style using the above as focus points.
7. Compare and contrast his or her preference with yours.

Visual Arts: Cultural and Personal Connections

1. If you were told today that you had a commendable amount of artistic talent, what visual or plastic art form would you choose to work in (water color, oils, charcoal, wood, clay, granite, etc.)?
2. What characteristics of this form would most influence your choice? What attracts you?
3. What style would you probably select (e.g., illustrative, representational, abstract, other)? What characteristics would most influence your choice?
4. What subject matter or theme would you probably choose? What factors would influence your choice?
5. Have you ever had or do you now have direct experience in the visual arts? If so, describe.

Continued on Page 136

ASSIGNMENTS, CONTINUED

Dance: Cultural and Personal Connections

1. Briefly identify the dance style with which you are most familiar.

2. How frequently do you participate in this dancing?

3. Describe your most familiar dance style. Include in this description consideration of
   - Sociocultural history and meaning
   - Rhythm and repetition
   - Movement and complexity (movement of the body, trunk, and extremities, fluidity, forcefulness, energy, etc.)
   - Skill required
   - Associated music
   - Interpersonal involvement

4. Interview an individual whose dance style is different from yours (e.g., an older adult, friend, or relative). Ask this person to describe his or her preferred and frequently used dance style using the above as focus points.

5. Compare and contrast his or her dance style with yours.

Drama: Cultural and Personal Connections

Briefly describe the type of drama you prefer and are involved with most frequently (e.g., stage plays, movies, television). In your description, include consideration and critique of
   - The main theme, the overall message, and focus of the dramas
   - Comedy or tragic orientation
   - Historical or current
   - Movement and speed of action
   - Fantasy or reality
   - Required acting skills
   - Size of cast
   - Complexity-simplicity of sets and/or filming

REFERENCES

Arieti, S. (1976). *Creativity: The magic synthesis*. New York: Basic Books.
Arnheim, R. (1969). *Visual thinking*. Berkeley, CA: University of California Press.
Bartenieff, I. (1980). *Body movement—Coping with the environment*. New York: Gordon & Breach.
Canaday, J. (1964). *Keys to art*. Paris: Fernand Hazen.
Griffiths, I. (1998, March 22). The thesis of music reflecting the culture of the times. *The New York Times*.
Hanna, J. L. (1987). *To dance is human: A theory of nonverbal communication*. Austin, TX: University of Texas Press.
Hanna, J. L. (1988). *Dance, sex, and gender*. Chicago: University of Chicago Press.
Hayman, D. (1969). *The arts and man*. New York: Prentice Hall.
Hermann, N. (1988). *The creative brain*. Lake Lure, NC: Brain Books.
Highwater, J. (1978). *Dance: Rituals of experience*. New York: Oxford University Press.
Hjort, M., & Laver, S. (1997). *Emotion and the arts*. New York: Oxford University Press.
Kosintsen, G. (1969). The cinema and our time. In: *The arts and man*. New York: Prentice Hall.
Laban, R. (1956). *Principles of dance and movement notation*. London: McDonald & Evans.
Lomax, A. (1968). *Folk song style and culture*. Washington, DC: American Association for the Advancement of Science.
Lomax, A., Bartenieff, I., & Paulay, F. (1968) Dance style and culture. In: A. Lomax. *Folk song style and culture*. Washington, DC: American Association for the Advancement of Science.
Marquet, J. (1986). *The aesthetic experiences*. New Haven, CT: Yale University Press.
Melnitz, W. (1969). The theatre and its continuing social function. In: d'Arcy Hayman. *Arts and man*. New York: Prentice Hall.
Menuhin, Y. (1969). Music and the nature of its contribution to humanity. In: d'Arcy Hayman. *Arts and man*. New York: Prentice Hall.
Nadeau, R. (1993). Using the visual arts to expand personal creativity. In: B. Warren. *Using the creative arts in therapy*. New York: Routledge.
Peloquin, S. M. (1996). Using the Arts to influence conflict learning. *Am J Occup Ther, 50*(2), 148-151.
Read, H. (1970). *Education through art*, 3rd ed. London: Farber & Farber.
Schiff, D. (1998, May 31). Classical radio plays only to sweet tooths.*The New York Times*.
Sommer, S. (1998, May 31). Hands dance, feet sing, and bodies are the drums. *The New York Times*.
Sparshott, F. (1997). *Emotions in theatre dance*. Princeton, NJ: Princeton University Press.
Warren, B. (1993). Using the imagination as a stepping stone for personal growth. In: B. Warren. *Using the creative arts in therapy*. New York: Routledge.
Warren, B., & Corten, R. (1993). Developing self image and self expression through movement. In: B. Warren. *Using the creative arts in therapy*. New York: Routledge.

ADDITIONAL READING

Aimes, H. T., Warren, B., & Watling, R. (1986). *Social drama*. London: John Clare Books.
Anderson, R. L. (1979). *Art in primitive societies*. Englewood Cliffs, NJ: Prentice Hall.
Brockert, O. G. (1974). *History of the theatre*, 2nd ed. Newton, MA: Allyn & Bacon.
Cunningham, M., & Lesschaeve, J. (1985). *The dancer and the dance*. New York: Marion Boyars.
Davies, S. (1994). *Musical meaning and expression*. Ithaca, NY: Cornell University Press.
Deway, J. (1934). *Art as experience*. New York: Pedigree.
Feder, E., & Feder, B. (1981). *The expressive arts therapies*. Sarasota, FL: Feder.
Goodman, N. (1976). *Language of art: An approach to a theory of symbolism*. Indianapolis: Hackett.
Hanna, J. L. (1983). *The performer-audience connection: Emotion to metaphor in dance and society*. Austin, TX: University of Texas Press.
Higgens, K. M. (1991). *The music of our lives*. Philadelphia: Temple University Press.
Janson, H. W. (1991). *History of art*. Englewood Cliffs, NJ: Prentice Hall.
Jung, C. G. (1966). *The spirit is man. Art and literature*. New York: Pantheon Books.
Keller, J. R., & Godbey, G. (1992). The arts as leisure. In: J. R. Keller & G. Godbey. *The sociology of leisure*. State College, PA: Venture Publishing Inc.
Kivy, P. (1990). *Music alone*. Ithaca, NY: Cornell University Press.
Lamb, W., & Watson, E. (1987). *Body code, The meaning in movement*. Princeton, NJ: Princeton Book Co.
Langer, S. (1953). *Feeling and town: A theory of art*. New York: Scribner.

Langon, S. (1976). *Philosophy in a new key. A study in the symbolism of reason, rite and art*, 3rd ed. Cambridge, MA: Harvard University Press.

Panosfsky, S. M. (1989). *Meaning in the visual arts*. Garden City, NJ: Doubleday/Anchor.

Sorell, W. (Ed.) (1966). *The dance has many faces*. New York: Columbia University Press.

Sparshott, F. (1982). *The theory of the arts*. Princeton, NJ: Princeton University Press.

Codes of Meaning: Jobs and Careers

Gail S. Fidler
Beth P. Velde

History teaches us that the very earliest division of labor was the result of the fundamental reality of women's ability to give birth and, thus, to carry responsibility for the feeding and care of the children. Because the men of the clan were not hearth bound, it was their responsibility to hunt and fish for the clans' food and to wage war in an effort to extent land to add to the food supply and to protect their territory. When farming was introduced, it was rational for the "home bound" women to take responsibility for planting and tending crops, as well as preparing the food and clothing and caring for the family.

The strength of such gender-based roles is vividly illustrated in the recent biography of Tecumseh (Sugden, 1998). It is conjectured that the demise of this wise and famous Indian chief was brought about by his refusal to enter into a compromise with the American government. A treaty would have seriously reduced the tribes' hunting and fishing land, forcing them to turn to farming for survival. Because the Indians firmly believed that farming was women's work, Tecumseh refused and chose to fight for the right of his warriors to hunt and fish.

In early pre-industrial societies, the tasks of survival and everyday living were woven into one. There was no distinction, as there is today, between work and leisure, no differentiation between what was essential and what was enjoyable. A symbiotic relationship existed between the people and nature (Kohn & Schooler, 1983). Nature held the power of life and death; the people held the challenge of survival, to overcome, placate, compromise, or outwit. The meaning of their daily life activities combined the instrumental realities with the symbolic messages of nurturing, caring, and growth, the arduous challenge of the hunt, shared relationships, and conquering or falling victim to the beauty and force of nature. Each task was integrally tied to the reality and symbol of the event. The values of a closely knit, mutually dependent agrarian society carried over into the early stages of the growth of guilds. Apprentices and masters shared in a man-to-man closeness, working and learning together. Csikszentmihalyi (1990) offers some intriguing, although at times somewhat biased, examples of the meaning of certain activities traditionally associated with daily living (pp. 144-154).

The industrial revolution brought about marked change in ways of living. The mechanized plow, the planter, and the harvester changed farming and the role of the farmer forever. Knitting machines and motor-propelled looms began to replace the hands of the weaver and knitter, significantly altering their role and the activity itself. In the previous chapter, it was suggested that there is a notably different experience between using one's voice as a music-producing instrument and manipulating an external instrument, such as violin or horn, to produce music. Can we make a similar claim here? Can we conjecture that to use one's hands or one's body to produce crops, clothing, food and/or tools is a neurophysiologically and psychologically different engagement, a qualitatively different sense of connectedness as compared with manipulating a machine in order to produce a product? How might the experiences be contrasted? What are the differences symbolically? As we noted earlier, a toy created by the child or pushed or moved by the hands and body of the child is an experience that contrasts with engagement and manipulation of a toy that is activated by a force external to the child. The industrial revolution also began to sharpen the distinction between men and women. Money gradually began to replace land as the basis and symbol of power. The men, as workers and wage earners, received the money and controlled the amount given to their mates. Thus, women became increasingly dependent on men for money.

As populations grew and society became more complex, there emerged greater demand for more and varied food, increased comforts, a greater variety of options, and more income to purchase these and sustain this new lifestyle. Jobs and careers began to be increasingly essential to daily living, but also more frequently less satisfying. As factories multiplied, end products began to be further and further removed from the process of creating them, with feedback and results less immediately related to one's effort. The assembly line became an institutionalized process and altered significantly the nature of performance and the meaning of the end products (Walker, 1957). A well-developed overview of the changes in patterns of daily living is provided in Wilcock's (1998) study of the evolution of occupation.

We have noted how the growing complexity of societies influenced and was reflected in a greater sophistication in styles of art, music, dance, and drama. A similar dynamic was played out in people's daily living activities. As industrialization spread, jobs and careers and their associated tasks became more specialized and diverse. This factor, along with the assembly line, created the need for an overseer, foreman, supervisor, and director. This complex music and orchestration required conductors! Furthermore, now, instead of the small-town farm and land, the corporation, "the industry," became the focal point, the core that held people together, the source of security, survival, identity, and community. The end product, the tasks that created it, and the environmental context of the process all came to symbolize these human needs and interests. In all probability, the auto industry has been the most notable example of this phenomena and Detroit a symbol of family, security, and belonging. This theme and its meaning are certainly evident in the traditional reference to AT&T as MaBell.

As the industrial era comes to a close, there have been and will continue to be marked changes again in the social order of things, in the environmental context of daily living, in the ways we identify and construct our lifestyle, and in the priority activities that will comprise that daily living. A current concern among young urban professionals is the lack of time and the increasing view of time as a commodity. As the pace of life accelerates, available time diminishes, and money is used to buy time for oneself. This may include, for instance, purchasing the time (service) of others to do one's yard work, clean the house, or prepare take-out meals. However, free time is not usually increased. There appears to be a pervasive attitude that if one is not engaged in something productive, one is not creating and defining self (Schor, 1991). The concepts of productive activity furthermore seems to have been extended to include the pursuit of leisure as well as work. And free time remains elusive. In addition, American corporations frequently see the amount of time spent on one's job as symbolic of the extent of an employee's commitment (Holt, Robinson, & Godbey, 1997).

The needs of an increasing aging population are giving impetus and extreme pressure to develop and expand a host of services related to special housing, community development, entertainment, and most certainly health care. The growth and mergers of banks, hospitals, and other corporations, and the break-up of industrial monopolies and downsizing of many others is altering how we define and operationalize many jobs, career functions, and skill expectations. Managed care has changed how health care is defined and how medicine and associated services are practiced. The computer has had an impact on almost every aspect of daily living. It has changed how we bank and manage our money, pay bills, work, make purchases, and plan trips and vacations. It has influenced how we view time, because it measures time in frames and spans impossible for the human to experience. Once individuals become acclimated to the speed of the computer, human social interaction seems laborious.

Technology has dramatically influenced how we perceive the workplace. In an increasingly competitive job market, employees find themselves extending the work site to the home, hotel, and airplane, for example. Lap-top computers, faxes, cellular phones, and modems all provide access to the job, 24 hours a day from virtually anywhere. *Fortune* magazine (February 24, 1997) reports that estimates suggest that each new home worker spends $3,000 to $5,000 to establish a home office and an additional $1,000 yearly for upgrades and supplies. Clearly, the physical separation of home and work appears to be decreasing. In addition to the business world, the changes in health care are increasingly changing one's work site from the hospital to care in the home.

Meanwhile, noteworthy change seems to be taking place in the corporate setting. Writing in *The New York Times*, Bryant (1998) describes some of the emerging policies that reflect changing perspectives regarding the purpose and meaning of work. Social and economic developments, such as continuing prosperity, negatives of the 1980s era's greed, and the aging and altered priorities of the baby boomers have all helped to generate a growing expectation that there should be more to a job or career than the paycheck. At the same time, companies reaching the limits of downsizing and reorganization are "coming to realize that one of the few remaining ways to get more out of workers is to help them find purpose. People are searching for meaning in the workplace and employers are happy to help them" (p. 1, sec. 4).

Current literature, numerous management books, and business journals emphasize that empowering is out and enabling is in. Companies are employing motivational consultants and speakers, offering classes in religion and educational topics, and granting paternity leave and other time-off opportunities as ways of responding to the family needs of workers. There seems to be a diminishing line between work and other aspects of daily living. The practice of participatory management in some forms may well be reemerging as the move grows to give workers a broader mission than taking home a paycheck. Bryant (1998) reminds us that J. Walch, the chairman of General Electric, has for several years extolled the value of a "boundaryless" workplace, where every one contributes to the entire organization rather than tending to his or her own turf.

Interpersonal values and attitudes certainly shape the nature and meaning of the work setting and the performance imperatives of a job or career. The emotional and interpersonal context has most characteristically been viewed as significant in those occupations concerned with addressing human needs. Thus, affective and interpersonal skills are more frequently expected and associated with, for example, careers in teaching, nursing, medicine, rehabilitation, business, and industry. Especially the corporate workplace has generally viewed such skills as not being a priority and frequently as counterproductive to management and high production levels. The affective, attitudinal, and interpersonal behaviors expected and required of a job or a career clearly help to create an environmental context, shape and define what engagement in a given job or career can mean, realistically and symbolically (Beck & Hillmar, 1986; Goleman, 1995; Kanter, 1983; Senge, 1995).

These alterations, the shifts in job, career, and education preferences, their redesign and reordering, the newly developing opportunities, and increased options are only a few examples of changing focus and service demands. The idea that careers, jobs, and even school subjects embody meaning well beyond their actual function is perhaps less readily understood than the role of the symbolic process in the creative arts. The symbolic meaning of culture is too frequently overlooked in the psychological sciences (Shweder & LeVine, 1984). Nevertheless, each of us has, on occasion, experienced a reaction to an event that suggests that we categorize or judge a given job or career according to criteria that is unrelated to its reality. For instance, we are startled to learn that Rosie Greer did needlepoint, that our auto mechanic has a PhD, that the ballet dancer races sports cars, or the surgeon weeps. Our expectation in developing this chapter is that taking a closer look at the evolution of meaning, coming to see the interrelationship of reality and symbolic thought, and assessing and comparing performance imperatives will lead to a broader understanding of the meaning of those activities that comprise a job, career, school subject, or volunteer undertaking.

The social and cultural significance of an occupation is directly related to the value that society places on that activity. Value is measured by the extent to which the occupation relates directly to the critical concerns, needs, and interests of society, the complexity of knowledge and/or skill required, and the demonstrated credibility of that occupation (i.e., its effectiveness in addressing concerns and needs that, in many instances, are manifested in earning power). As the needs and interests of society change, so does the significance or status of a given job or career. Applying this criteria, one might conclude that the job of a Maytag repairman was on the brink of extinction, while the significance and relevance of the computer instructor and programmer is spiraling to impressive heights. As recently as 10 or more years ago, for example, entering politics and gaining a congressional seat carried with it status and prestige. Today, the public questions about the government's credibility has significantly lowered the status of this occupation. Twenty or more years ago, the stature and credibility of certain medical specialties were different than they are today. In years past, psychiatry, for example, occupied a position near the top of the list of preferred specialties. Today, it rates a significantly lower position on the list. Society decreed that deinstitutionalization and the resulting street people demonstrated psychiatry's failure to cure mental illness, and its credibility eroded. By contrast, physical medicine was relatively unknown and, accordingly, was low on the list of popular specialties. However, the extreme popularity of sports and, thus, sports medicine today has moved physical medicine to near the top among credible specialties.

The significance accorded jobs and careers by society has an important role in shaping their symbolic and actual meaning. Society determines and rewards those occupations deemed capable of addressing its important concerns, needs, and interests. Throughout history, those roles that encompass responsibilities or functions that deal with the life and death concerns of a society embody forceful meaning (Etzioni, 1969). From primitive medicine man, shaman, priest, and mother to modern day physician, theologian, nurse, mother, and lawyer, there are the continuing associations with healing, care, nurturance, protection and eternal life. It does not, therefore, require a stretch of the imagination to understand the reverence accorded the practice of law that prevents the death penalty, the surgery that saves a life, the nursing care that sustains it, or the theology that ensures personal peace, serenity, and a life after death.

In addition to the importance of addressing life and death issues as a dynamic force in ascribing meaning, there is the relevance of skill in determining both real and symbolic value. Job skills are frequently categorized to include the cognitive domain of problem identification and solution, judgment, manual manipulation, physical skills, and people and psychological skills (Kohn & Schooler, 1983). There is a hierarchical ordering of jobs and careers, and the familiar phrase "up the corporate ladder" clearly expresses this reality. Jobs and careers are rated in part by the complexity of the skills they require, the degree of supervision they require, and the extent of decision-making freedom and responsibility they entail. Obviously, the greater complexity and diversity of the skills required in a given job or career, the greater is the respect and value accorded by society. The validity of this equation is evident, for example, in the respect accorded careers in nuclear physics, aerospace, medicine, law, and computer science. The career of the professional athlete of today is a further example of societies' keen interest in competitive sports, high respect for uncommon skill and the revenues generated combine to create hero worship. The real and inferred messages that relate to the value and significance of cognitive skills are clear—the instant wealth and influence of the computer scientist. The computer as a way of life, as the pathway into the internal and external world of self and others, to a virtual reality, has created a sense of magic and virtual self-agency, an intelligence that has transformed perspectives, real and imagined.

In contrast, those jobs and careers that, in the recent past, have been the responsibility of the family or other citizens of a community are frequently viewed as requiring fewer skills and less complexity. They are, therefore, accorded more limited status and rewards than the unordinary, more complex occupations. Examples have included those careers related to parenting and daily living concerns, such as child care, care of the aged or disabled, housekeeping, nursing, and kindergarten schooling. We are well aware of the teaching profession's long struggles over many decades to gain heightened credibility and status. To alter the sociocultural meaning of an occupation requires time and persistent public education and demonstration in order for society to understand the complexity and diversity of the skills required in many of these careers.

One additional dimension of cultural symbolism and meaning is the gender-specific orientation that characterizes certain occupations (Brown, 1970). For centuries, those daily living activities concerned with nurturance, care and feeding, birthing, and the laying on of hands have been understood as the primary role and responsibility of women, while those tasks and activities with characteristics similar to the early roles of hunter, fisherman, and warrior have traditionally been regarded as the domain of men. Thus, jobs and careers that emphasize strength, aggression, endurance, force, calculation and strategy, and literal or symbolic warfare have traditionally been acknowledged as male occupations. Although a number of significant changes are currently challenging our stereotyping, the real and symbolic values and beliefs that comprise meaning are deeply ingrained in all societies.

While technology has significantly reduced the strenuous demands of housework, it does not appear to have decreased the amount of time or breadth of activities of the job. All indications seem to reflect an agreement that the time required to fulfill housekeeping duties has not been reduced significantly. Furthermore, the view of these activities as not constituting "work" continues. The phrase, "the nonworking mother or housewife," seems as ubiquitous as ever. From the very earliest social grouping to the present day, the belief that women's place is in the home has continued to hold strong value in society. As the number of women in the workforce continues its dramatic growth, the conflicts and ambiguities created by these realities continue to plague society.

How the duties and responsibilities of housework are defined and symbolically expressed varies according to socioeconomic and political contexts. For example, during the mid 1900s, the station wagon symbolized an important duty of the privileged, suburban, middle-class housewife. The vehicle was for carpooling, trips to dancing class, softball and field hockey practice, and scouts, etc. Today, it has been replaced by the minivan, but the symbols and rituals continue. The crowded local family restaurants on a Thursday night signaled the maids day off, symbolizing a certain economic level and definition of housekeeping tasks and responsibilities. The sight of the laundry truck and clothes drying on the line or in the laundromat are further examples of the variations in job description of housekeeping. A comparable example of today's variations can perhaps be demonstrated by a cook in the kitchen, carry-out dinners, fast food drive-ins, or frozen meals from the supermarket. Buying the time of others to fulfill housekeeping duties obviously shapes the nature and meaning of the job in ways that contrast with total responsibility for all tasks and duties. The nature of the job varies according to the ability or willingness to pay others to fulfill one's tasks.

Child care has always been understood to be an inherent and significant aspect of housewife responsibilities. It is, then, in some ways, an important part of the job of working in the house. In many decades past, such responsibilities included the education of the children as well as full care for their total daily activities. The advent of kindergarten, nursery schools, and infant and child care centers have resulted in children spending significant time away from home, early in their lives. Most frequently, the child benefits from learning experiences in different interpersonal and physical environments. However, the availability and quality of such experiences varies according to socioeconomic and political factors.

The transfer of a portion of child care to people and settings outside of the home alters the nature of the job duties of housewife and mother. Society's ambivalence about the woman's place in the home or workforce gets played out in many ways that have an impact on how this job is perceived and defined.

Early in the 20th century, the manufacturers of household products became aware of the housewife and her housekeeping activities as a rich source of potential revenue. Germ-free homes were promoted as the goal of every responsible, credible housewife. Lysol products waged germ warfare to achieve a germ-free home. Cleaning products made it possible to achieve floors so shiny as to reflect the very character of the housewife (Ewen, 1976). The force of such advertising continues to warn against ring-around-the-collar, dull white clothes, and numerous other threatening oversights of the careless housekeeper. All of these messages infer and symbolically reflect a high standard of performance and expectations regarding the role and responsibility of respectable housekeeping. The pressures to comply and the increased time that was necessary to meet such standards and other responsibilities of the job created both stress and ambivalence (Schor, 1991). Although the squeaky-clean house of a generation or two is less of a model today, this ethic has been well internalized and influences, in many ways, how the job or career of housekeeping is perceived and what it means both realistically and symbolically.

- *What jobs and/or careers can you identify as reflecting one or more of those characteristics that have been discussed?*
- *How might the relationship between the characteristics of this occupation and its sociocultural meaning be explained?*
- *How has society's perception of this occupation changed?*
- *How would you characterize your profession?*
- *Which characteristic seems most significant in defining the meaning of this career?*

Although the sociocultural identity of a given occupation is critical to understanding its full meaning, this dimension does not tell the entire story. Factual and subjective meaning are very much related to the performance requirements of a job or career. The action processes and concomitant objects of a given occupation are imbued with realistic and symbolic meaning. To understanding meaning, it is imperative that those action processes, the performance imperatives that define an occupation, be assessed.

Analyzing and interpreting the findings of a 20-year study developed to assess the impact of social structure on personality, Kohn and Schooler (1983) produced a viable format for assessing both the structural and performance imperatives of a given occupation. Using the *Dictionary of Occupational Titles* as an organizational guide, these researchers produce guidelines for the classification of the complexity of a given occupation. This classification addresses levels of performance complexity relative to the management of data, of things (objects), and of people. A final overall complexity assessment offers a guide for summarizing the cognitive or intellectual demands of an occupation on a seven-point rating scale. The structural imperatives that are defined in this work address what might be called the environmental context. Factors in this category involve evaluations of the amount of self-direction versus amount of supervision, job pressures, job security, and position in the organizational structure. It is evident that exploration of the dimensions of each of these elements is an essential process in reaching an understanding of the nature and meaning of a job or career.

An indispensable perspective regarding the performance imperatives will be gained by examining the neurophysiological and psychologically based functions that are necessary in a given occupation. In his description of how cultural competence is transmitted, Gardner (1986) identifies seven forms of information processing. Each of these addresses a competency that can readily be understood as relevant to job or career performance and can be related to as supplementing Kohn's and Schooler's classifications. The seven forms offered by Gardner include the following:

- *Linguistic competencies:* language skills, such as those required of journalists, writers, public speakers.

- *Spatial competence:* the capacity of one's nervous system to discern visual patterns and depth elements, the spatial intelligence required of architect, artist, engineer, and physicist.

- *Logical, mathematical competence:* the capacity to enumerate elements and see cause-and-effect relationships, which are necessary for mathematical and scientific careers, such as researchers and accountants.

- *Kinesthetic competence:* the capacity to carry out complex motor patterns, those skills required by the athlete, hunter, dancer, craftsman.

- *Musical competence:* a highly tuned auditory system, sensitivity to tone and pitch. This competency is related in part to linguistic skill and mathematical ability and, of course, is primarily evident in all aspects of music careers.

- *Interpersonal competence:* social and interpersonal skills, awareness of others. An essential requirement of the helping professions, such as social work, ministry, nursing, and counseling.

- *Intrapersonal or personal competence:* knowledge and awareness of self, a sensitivity to one's own needs, interests, and motivations, a sense of self-identity and executive function. Especially relevant for successful performance in the helping careers, the performing arts, and as manager, director, and planner.

Using these forms of information processing in conjunction with the activity analysis presented in Chapter 6 will expand the understanding of the innate characteristics and performance requirements of a given job or career.

These competencies call to mind the studies and research devoted to the structure and neurophysiology of the brain. Spurred by the split brain surgeries of the 1960s, the explosion of studies and publications in the past decade related to brain functions has been and continues to be impressive. The work of Hermann (1988) is, at this time, most directly relevant to the focus of this chapter. His principle interest and concern is to relate certain brain structures and functions to the unique characteristics of jobs and careers and to styles of learning.

Hermann's studies have shown that, in the brain's left hemisphere, the cerebral or upper lobe contains those processes that comprise technical, analytical, mathematical, logical, and problem-solving behaviors. The lower left lobe or left limbic lobe houses those processes that are controlled, conservative, and concerned with planning and organizing. His research has, furthermore, demonstrated that these functions are predominant in jobs and careers related to the practice of medicine (except for psychiatry), law, engineering, banking, science, investment, accounting, book-keeping, management, administration, and other occupations requiring logical, analytical, quantitative, fact-based, planned, organized, detailed, and sequential behaviors.

In the right hemisphere of the brain, the cerebral or upper lobe houses the artistic, holistic, flexible, imaginative, and synthesizing processes. The lower, limbic lobe of the right hemisphere is the source of emotional, spiritual, musical, interpersonal, and empathic processes. It has been shown that these processes are most evident in those jobs or careers of the teacher, nurse (except nurse administrator), musician, artist, dancer, social worker, psychiatrist, clergy, entrepreneur, and in other occupations that require holistic, intuitive, synthesizing, integrating, interpersonal, kinesthetic, and feeling-based behaviors.

This very condensed and limited ordering certainly does not do justice to Hermann's work. It is only the very tip of the iceberg of his intriguing and complex constructs. What we have presented here should stimulate further study in the relationship between job performance imperatives and brain function, thus, enhancing our appreciation of meaning. Hermann's *The Creative Brain* (1988) should be a priority resource in the teaching-learning process of those whose careers relate to teaching, management, counseling, and most certainly rehabilitation.

The myriad meanings associated with jobs and careers and their impressive complexity cannot possibly be adequately explored here. We can only expect to trigger awareness and stimulate a continuing study. The following assignments have been planned to engage the student in further exploration of the tip of this very large iceberg.

The Interview Guide: Primary Occupation, appearing at the end of this chapter, provides an outline to guide the development of a description of a person's primary occupation. The student is asked to write a description of his or her current or most recent job or career, using the outline as a guide. If the student has never been employed, a volunteer responsibility could be used instead, or the role of student within a chosen career can be used as the primary occupation.

When this career description has been completed, it is expected that small discussion groups will be formed to compare and contrast descriptions, to describe similarities and differences, and to arrive at some overall observations based on comparisons.

When this assignment is completed, the student is asked to interview a person (not a student) using the outline as a guide. Following the write-up of the interview, small discussion groups should reconvene to compare and contrast the occupational histories that have been obtained to compare these with their own and develop some generalizations about similarities and differences.

Interview Guide: Primary Occupation

The term *primary occupation* refers to those activities that occupy the majority of an individual's time and attention and are related to earning an income and/or meeting the physical needs and welfare of others. It encompasses those activities that relate to social obligation (i.e., job, career, educational, or volunteer pursuits).

1. Describe your primary occupation.
2. What influenced your occupational choice?
3. What is the most enjoyable aspect for you?
4. What do you like least about it?
5. Which aspects of your occupation are the easiest for you to manage?
6. Which ones are the most difficult?
7. What skills do you have that are important to your occupation?
8. To what extent do you enjoy what you are doing?
9. Describe the kind of person you think it takes to do well in your kind of occupation.
10. How well do you fit that profile?
11. What are the most important characteristics of your occupation?
12. How would you describe your occupation in terms of its:
    - Complexity
    - Supervision
    - Routines and detail
    - Pressures
    - Security
    - Compensations (such as money, awards, time, etc.)
    - Status
13. How important do you think your occupation is to society?
14. If you could change your occupational choice, what changes would you make?
15. What hobbies and related free-time activities do you regularly engage in?
16. How are these different from your primary occupation?
17. Considering all aspects, what does your occupation mean to you?

REFERENCES

Beck, A. C., & Hillmar, E. D. (1986). *Positive management practices*. San Francisco: Jossey Bass.

Bridges, W. (1994, February 24). The end of the job. *Fortune*. p. (from beth).

Brown, J. K. (1970). A note on the division of labor by sex. *American Anthropologist, 72,* 1073-1078.

Bryant, A. (1998). Quest for fire. *The New York Times*, section 4, p. 1.

Campbell, B. G. (1988). *Humankind emerging*. New York: Harper Collins.

Csikszentmihalyi, M. (1990). *Flow: The psychology of optimal experiences*. New York: Harper & Row.

Etzioni, A. (Ed.). (1969). *The semi-professional: Teachers, nurses, social workers*. New York: The Free Press.

Ewen, S. (1976). *Captains of consciousness: Advertising and the social roots of consumer culture*. New York: McGraw-Hill.

Gardner, H. (1986). Culture theory: The development of competence in culturally defined domains. In: R. Shueder & R. LeVine. *Culture theory essays on mind, self, and emotion*. New York: Cambridge University Press.

Goleman, D. (1995). *Emotional intelligence*. New York: Bantam Books.

Hermann, N. (1988). *The creative brain*. Lake Lure, NC: Brain Books, Inc.

Holt, H., Robinson, J. D., & Godbey, G. (1997). *Time for life: The surprising ways Americans use time*. State College, PA: Pennsylvania State University Press.

Kanter, R. M. (1983). *The change masters*. New York: Simon & Schuster.

Kohn, W., & Schooler, C. (1983). *Work and personality*. Norwood, NJ: Ablex Publishing Co.

Schor, J. B. (1991). *The overworked Americans*. New York: Basic Books.

Senge, P. (1995). *The fifth discipline*. San Francisco: Jossey Bass.

Shweder, R. A., & LeVine, R. A. (1984). *Culture theory*. New York: Cambridge University Press.

Sugden, J. (1998). *Tecumseh*. New York: Harry Holt & Co.

Walker, C. R. (1957). *Toward the automatic factory: A case study of men and machines*. New Haven, CT: Yale University Press.

Wilcock, A. A. (1998). *An occupational perspective of health*. Thorofare, NJ: SLACK, Incorporated.

ADDITIONAL READING

Bernard, J. (1981). *The female world*. New York: Free Press.

Hochschild, A. R. (1997). *The timebind: When work becomes home and home becomes work*. New York: Henry Holt.

Inglehart, R. (1990). *Culture shift in industrial society*. Princeton, NJ: Princeton University Press.

Kelly, J. R., & Godbey, G. (1992). *The sociology of leisure*. State College, PA: Ventura Press.

Lee, R. B., & DeVore, I. (1968). *Man the hunter*. Chicago: Aldine Publishing Company.

LeGoft, C. (1980). *Time, work and culture in the middle ages*. Chicago: University of Chicago Press.

Leider, R. (1997). *Power of purpose: Creating meaning in your life and work*. New York: Berrett Koehler.

Nippert, E. C. (1995). *Home and work: Negotiating boundaries through every day life*. Chicago: University of Chicago.

Peters, T. (1997). *Circle of innovation*. New York: Knopf.

Rifkin, J. (1987). *The primary conflict in human history*. New York: Tarcher-Putnam.

Rifkin, J. (1995). *The end of work*. New York: Putnam.

Super, D. E. (1957). *The psychology of careers*. New York: Harper Collins.

Terkel, S. (1972). *Working*. New York: Avon.

Thompson, E. P. (1963). *The making of the English working class*. New York: Viking Press.

Treiman, D. J. (1977). *Occupational prestige in comparative perspective*. New York: Academic Press.

Vroom, V. H. (1995). *Work and motivation*. San Francisco: Jossey-Bass, Inc.

Wilensky, H. (1960). Work, careers and social integration. *International Social Science Journal, 12,* 543-560.

Messages of the Environment

Gail S. Fidler

There is a wealth of information dealing with the environment as a forceful influence on behavior and on the shaping of attitudes and values. These ever-expanding bodies of knowledge have had a marked impact on, for example, community planning, education, business and industry, and health systems. Along with a growing sophistication regarding the relevance of the environment in all aspects of human performance, there has evolved a change in the definition of the term. Earlier perspectives viewed the environment as referencing physical elements, such as structural design, space, light, temperature, accessibility, furnishings, and safety. More recently, psychological and sociological factors have been recognized as critical aspects of an environment. This broader concept includes, for example, consideration of group formations, social networking, person-to-person relationships, emotional tone, eating patterns, and cognitive expectations. What has emerged is the concept of environmental context. Several commendable, brief overviews of environmental studies related to occupational therapy have been published recently. These and their reference listings, especially, offer relevant background material for this chapter (Corcoran & Gitlin, 1997; Dunn, Brown, & McGuigan, 1994; Fidler, 1996; Spencer, 1991).

Because the theme of this text is the meaning of activities, the intent in developing this chapter is to limit our focus to looking at the role and influence of activities in both shaping and reflecting an environmental context. Our concern is to identify and examine the routines, tasks, and activities that comprise environmental components. Then, we will consider these from the perspective of how they convey, shape, and reflect attitudes, values, and performance expectations, as well as how they define the nature of human relationships and behaviors. More explicitly, this exploration will look at the dynamics of some of the ways in which the components of the environment encourage, support, or preclude certain activities as well as the ways that activities determine the nature of the environmental context. This focus represents a somewhat unique and narrow aspect of environmental study. Consequently, literature that is relevant to this theme is limited and frequently obscure. This reality means that, at times, we are exploring virgin territory as we seek to bridge activity characteristics to environmental characteristics.

Spencer (1991) calls attention to the work of Spivak (1973) and his coining of the term "archetypal places." He has described settings of the physical environment, such as spaces and furnishings, that support and make possible fundamental human activities, such as sleeping, grooming, eating, and working. Spencer suggests that this thesis at least infers an inherent connection between space and patterns of activity. In support of this theme, it is noted that there are special aspects of the environment that exist in response to human survival needs, such as the grocery stores, pharmacies, restaurants, and the like. There are also those spaces that make it possible for individuals to attend to emotional needs, such as churches, parks, museums, wooded paths, lakes, and mountain peaks. Our pursuit of a deeper understanding of activities leads us to then ask questions such as what is the nature of those activities that characteristically occur in these places? In what ways do these activities shape and create the culture of the setting? What behavioral expectations are communicated by the space?

Obviously, there are numerous and varied groups and individual activities associated with each of these places. Traditionally, however, these activities of personal care, subsistence, and pleasure have been studied from the perspective of person-activity relevance. The activity-environment dynamic has seldom been a priority for study. Kelly and Godbey (1992) warn that when one's perspective is focused on what people do without consideration of the environment, the context of the doing, the critical symbiotic relationship between the two, is ignored. They emphasize that what people do and how they do it is influenced by the environment and, in turn, impacts the environment.

The importance of space in terms of human activity was also explored by Hall (1966). He looked at the dimensions of space in terms of distance and closeness and the nature of interpersonal engagement that seemed to be stimulated or inhibited by varying distances between people. Furthermore, he compared and contrasted differing cultural patterns related to the meaning of spatial distance and closeness. This research showed that different cultures define interpersonal space differently. Perkins and Shoemaker (1990) report a correlation between the behaviors of children and space in school and the play environment. They were able to link open space to large motor activities and group clusters, and they linked limited, restricted space to more individual, intimate, and reflective activities.

Moving from consideration of space, Spencer (1991) directs her overview to aspects of the environment that relate to interior design and furnishings. What we find here that is relevant to our focus is the concept of cues. There is evidence that objects and furnishings trigger certain behaviors. Individuals behave differently when certain objects are part of their environment (Barker, 1963). This should not be a surprise after our study about objects in Chapter 4. Furnishings and other objects do indeed cue certain behaviors and infer or signal what kinds of activity are expected in a given setting. For example, the space and furnishings of a church or a temple set quite clear expectations for what activities, symbolic rituals, and behaviors are natural and appropriate in that space. Likewise, a ball field, gymnasium, library, or concert hall send silent messages, spark certain behaviors, and make possible, perhaps even demand, certain activities.

Corcoran and Gitlin (1997) note that natural and constructed objects support the rituals and routine activities of everyday life. Corroborating the findings of others, these authors emphasize the significance of furnishings and other objects in sustaining culturally derived rituals and everyday habits and routines. People design their surroundings to make a statement about themselves. And the design of their space and the objects that are displayed indicate the kinds of activities that take place in that setting as well as support and sustain those activities. For instance, a living space in which a piano and books of music are the focal point of a room certainly reflects the kind of activities most likely to occur and be encouraged in that space. Similarly, what messages are sent and what activities are supported when a classroom is furnished with student work tables set in small circles with a diversity of many objects and materials available throughout the area? What would probably be the nature of activities that take place in a classroom where student desks are set in rows, supply cabinets are closed and locked, and a book shelf is neatly arranged with several reference books?

Time plays a unique role in the environment. In addition to mechanical time usually measured by the clock, temporal elements of the environment also include social time, natural time, and biological time. In early history, before the advent of a device for measuring time, time itself may have been experienced more holistically. The time it took to complete an activity was dependent upon the interrelationship of the activity, the environmental requirements of the activity, and the motivation of the person. Since the advent of time-measuring devices, mechanical time has been measured in various units. These units have been somewhat arbitrarily divided into periods of time that often determine the type of activity that occurs. With the advent of the computer, these units have become smaller and smaller. Man's experiencing of time stress is usually equated to a real or perceived lack of mechanical time in which to accomplish the required activities for everyday living.

Social time is identified by social customs and rituals. For example, it is easy to identify lunchtime and the end of work time in the workplace, the end of class time on college campuses, the end of the school day at the local high school, or bedtime. Yet, this time is somewhat artificially regulated and controlled by customs of the predominant culture and is linked intimately with both the real and symbolic meaning of activities. Examples in this category might also include meal times in the home, family television watching, and happy hour after work.

Natural time is also referred to as cyclic time. It is the time that recurs across night and day, throughout the seasons, and within the lunar cycles. It is also linked realistically and symbolically to activity. Each fall, bonfires burn; each spring, new gardens are planted. Activities are governed by time of day. Outdoor, physical activities are conducted during the early morning and late afternoon hours, away from the heat of the day. Older adults may prefer activities occurring during the daylight, when decreased vision does not interfere with enjoyment or safety.

Biological time refers to the biological rhythms. These include the infradian rhythms (those that are longer than a day, such as women's menstrual periods), circadian rhythms (those that rise and fall once each day, such as the sleep/wake cycle), and ultradian rhythms (periods of activity alternated with periods of rejuvenation). While individuals vary in how they experience these biological rhythms, it is widely accepted that they do affect people and their engagement in activities. The physical environment is often designed to accommodate people's biological rhythms. Increasingly, activities are scheduled so they might occur to maximize participation and enjoyment based upon an individual's biological time. What additional examples of each of these can be offered from your own experience?

Addressing the significance of the environment within institutions, Fidler and Bristow (1992) remind us again that the design and use of space can create social and psychological barriers or it can foster social interaction and collaborative behaviors. The design and arrangement of furnishings within a space, they contend, can distance people from one another, emphasize privacy, separateness, and solo activity. This sense or distance is epitomized in institutions by long, unbroken corridors, chairs arranged in lines against the walls, and closed doors and partitions that separate areas of a room. By contrast, furniture arranged in small clusters or circles, open doors, and congregate space encourage face-to-face encounters and activities of interaction. The environmental context of facilities and institutions is described as including two interacting dimensions. These are expressed as the interpersonal structures and procedures, these human aspects of operations, and, secondly, the physical qualities of architectural design, routines, and schedules, the non-human dimensions of operations. The activities that comprise the essence of each of these are symbolic statements about the values, attitudes, and beliefs that characterize the institution and the home. Fidler and Bristow (1992) give an account of how these were played out in one particular setting, and in so doing they provide a stimulus for learning more about the relationships between activities and the environment.

Much has been written about the workplace environment and its impact on worker productivity. Peters and Waterman (1982), for example, addressed the relationship between a company's environment, its culture, and its performance. The processes for creating an environment that is responsive to the needs and interests of employees has been a prominent focus of most management texts for many years (Beck & Hillmar, 1986; Bolman & Deal, 1984; Hersey & Blanchard, 1982; Kanter, 1983; Senge, 1990). Furthermore, there seems to be a consensus among the experts about which human needs should be acknowledged and responded to by management practices. Studies have confirmed that successful, productive businesses and industries regularly provide a range of activities that address the needs of employees. Included are those management-supported activities that relate to the workers' need to achieve a sense of competence, to be acknowledged for achievement, to affiliate with others, to feel safe and secure, to achieve a measure of self-esteem, and to have evidence of being able to influence the important events of their lives. Therefore, frequently relevant activities within an organization include awards ceremonies and other celebrations that recognize and honor competence and achievement; holiday and social events that bring employees and management together; as well as various standing committees with full or partial worker membership that, for example, plan, manage, or monitor such functions as safety, finances, quality control, and trouble shooting. A family's culture is also defined through activities. These tend to center around the celebration of birthdays, special achievements of a family member, parties that connect with friends and neighbors, family outings, vacations and special trips, attendance at community events, game playing, religious observance, holiday celebrations, and involvement with school and church.

Bolman and Deal (1984) presented an intriguingly provocative thesis related to the symbolism that is involved in certain organizational cultures and rituals. Their construct has some relevance to our study of activities and reinforces the concept of meaning beyond what is obvious and manifest. Most among us, at one time or another, have sensed and noted that a given organizational activity was more symbolic than real. Perhaps the most ubiquitous example is "the team." Other activities that, at times, seem mostly symbolic include the endless committee meetings that lead only to more meetings or the task forces whose reports are filed for later consideration. Bolman and Deal (1984) contend that, frequently, who belongs to a committee is more important than what goes on within that committee. What is usually most important, they suggest, is not what really happened in a given event but the meaning of what happened. These authors, as part of their study of organizational management, explore the symbolic dimensions of the culture and the environmental context of organizations.

An environment is created by the interactive dimensions of interpersonal, social, cultural, temporal, and physical elements. The challenge at this point in our study is to attempt to concertize these elements in order to identify and describe those activities that are an inherent part of each. This endeavor should then make it possible to assess and study the activity aspects of a given environment and to ultimately relate these to universal human needs.

Because environments are complex, the task of environmental assessment is complex and difficult. Those assessments that have been standardized are mostly limited to one aspect, such as the design of space, social elements, or specialized settings. Letts, Law, Rigby, et al (1994) have published a listing of 41 assessments that incorporate concepts of person-environment fit. Each of these is considered in terms of its purpose, applicability, and reliability. This information is a valuable resource for selecting an appropriate, specialty-focused assessment. However, assessments and guidelines for exploring and studying the activity aspects of an environment have yet to be developed. It seems reasonable, nevertheless, to conjecture that if the principle components of an environment can be identified and described, if those activities that shape and reflect each component can likewise be identified and described, then such descriptive material should offer some reliable evidence of those environmental activities that address fundamental human needs.

The following nine environmental components are identified as characterized by certain activities that help to shape, support, and reflect the meaning of the component. As each one of these is defined and examined, the questions to be addressed include

- What activities actually comprise this component?
- Who are the persons involved?
- What symbolic culture and ritual is evident?
- What is the frequency of the activities?

Time management: Activities that relate to the development, disbursement, and monitoring of schedules, procedures, time, and structure of the rhythm of the day. The groups and committees that determine and schedule holiday celebrations and special events. Activities that comprise social, natural, and biologic time.

Space: Those activities that relate to the allocation of space. The impact of spatial design and allocation of activities, such as committee meetings, task forces, social events, informal meetings, daily routines, and privacy.

Facility and home management: The major tasks and activities that are related to maintenance of physical spaces, such as cleaning, trash removal, bed making, lighting, heating, safety, care of furnishings, and care of grounds.

Furnishings: Activities concerned with the purchase and use of furnishings and activities that are encouraged and supported or excluded by the types of furnishings; groups and activities responsible for the arrangement of areas.

Food: Activities related to the planning, selection, preparation, serving, eating, and clean-up of food, task forces, groups, and/or committees concerned with planning food and menus for special events and eliciting member or employee preferences.

Communication: Those activities that are part of the communication process. Committees, clusters, or group activities related to gathering, publishing, and disseminating information, such as newsletters, flyers, official documents, small and large group discussions, lectures, etc.

Decision making: Committee, group, or individual activities that discuss, critique, and make or recommend decisions. Activities of a family council or caucus, for example, or student government, advisory boards, board of directors, executive council, and union representative groups.

Affiliation: Activities that signify inclusion and belonging, such as formal and informal groups that plan and carry out special ceremonies and events, team sports, creation and display of the company logo and similar identity objects, T-shirts, health care, investment and retirement services, group trips, picnics, and retreats. Activities that connect with the outside community, such as church affiliations, public education programs, community services, volunteering, and other contributions.

Individualization: Activities that encourage and support individuality, that differentiate the individual from the total group, that reward individual initiative, such as planned celebrations of citizen of the year award, employee of the month, honor roll achievement, team leader, winning gold stars, gaining special privileges, life review groups, show and tell, talent shows, creating scrapbooks and photo albums, and displaying trophies, awards, and diplomas.

I have proposed that an environment will maximize individual performance to the extent that it includes and emphasizes those activities, those doing experiences, that address fundamental human needs (Fidler, 1996). This proposition suggests a relationship between the characteristics of certain environmental activities and the following human needs, which are reprinted from Fidler (1996):

- *Autonomy*: to be self-determining, gain a sense of being in control of one's life, and to be as self-dependent as personal needs and capacities define.

- *Individuality*: to be self-differentiating, to see and know one's uniqueness, to verify the existence and identity of oneself, distinguish self from others, and confirm the entitlement of one's interests, skills, and differences.

- *Affiliation*: to have evidence of belonging; be part of a dyad, group, or cluster; have associations with others; and know interdependence.

- *Volition*: to have alternatives, access to sufficient information, and latitude to make and act on one's choice.

- *Consensual validation*: to have feedback from one's activity and from other people that verify one's perceptions and reality and to be part of reciprocal exchanges that clarify and acknowledge one's contributions and actions.

- *Predictability*: to discern and evaluate cause and effect, be able to predict, limit ambiguity and chanciness, give order to one's world, and experience the comfort of predictability.

- *Self-efficacy*: to have evidence of one's competence, of being able to cope and manage one's everyday life, of being a cause, and of making things happen.

- *Adventure*: to seek and try out the new, the unknown; to explore; to look beyond the here and now; and to discover, experiment, and dare to risk.

- *Accommodation:* to be free from physical and mental harm and to function in an environment that is responsive to individual capabilities while compensating for individual limitations.

- *Reflection*: to have respite from activity, ponder on the meaning of things, and review and contemplate recent and past events.

It should now be possible to undertake an environmental assessment that will produce a profile of the components of an environment and related activities. Such a profile should make it feasible to then hypothesize about the relationship of such activities to basic human needs.

Using *The Environmental Context—Part I,* appearing at the end of this chapter, the first assignment is to assess and evaluate the environment of one's own home. Small group discussions should follow this assignment. The focus of this discussion is to critique the evaluation and data-gathering processes and compare and contrast the differences and similarities of findings and evaluative summaries.

Following this discussion, *The Environmental Context—Part II* should be completed, thus relating the characteristics of the environment that have been evaluated to the human needs listed in part II of the environmental context. The small discussion groups should then discuss and critique findings and offer some generalized summary constructs.

A second evaluative survey should be conducted involving either a school setting, a continued care facility, or a work setting. The same procedures should be followed as the ones applied to the evaluation of a home setting.

The information gathered from an activity-based environmental assessment not only provides a viable profile of an environment but, in a significant way, makes it possible to relate environmental activities to the human need responsiveness of a given environment. Such an equation, even with all of its imprecisions, enriches our understanding of the nature and meaning of activities, as well as the dynamics of the environmental context.

THE ENVIRONMENTAL CONTEXT—PART I

You are asked to identify and briefly describe the major activities that comprise a given environment. Your description is to focus on those activities, tasks, and routines that comprise the following environmental components, addressing the "what," the "when," and "by whom" for each.

Time management: Activities that involve the preparation and follow through of schedules and routine procedures. Those daily routines that form and sustain the rhythm of the day. Activities that comprise social, natural, and biologic time.

Food: Those activities related to the selection, preparation, serving, and eating of food and the clean-up that follows.

Communication: Those activities that comprise the processing and exchange of information, that establish, maintain, and define communication patterns.

Maintenance: The tasks and activities that attend to the routine maintenance of home or facility, those concerned with cleanliness, orderliness, and safety.

Decision making: Those activities that relate to and/or are a part of decision-making processes to include the levels at which such activities occur and the kind of decisions made.

Furnishings and possessions: The influence of the furnishings on activities, those that are encouraged or discouraged by the kind of furnishings, and their placement.

Space: Activities concerned with the allocation and organization of space. Those activities that are supported or precluded because of space. Spatial influence on the principle activities of the home or facility. Allocation of space for privacy.

Affiliation: Those activities that generate and sustain, relating associating and belonging among members. Those activities that members do together as well as those that connect the home or facility to the outside community.

Individualization: Activities that enable support and reward individual initiatives, that differentiate individual from the group and/or membership at large.

The Environmental Context—Part II

It has been hypothesized that human performance and the quality of life are enhanced in an environment that ensures including those doing experiences, those activities, that relate to the following 10 elements (Fidler, 1996).

A. Given the information you have gathered from your environmental activities assessment, how would you describe this environment in terms of each of these:

- *Autonomy:* to be self-determining, gain a sense of being in control of one's life, and be as self-dependent as personal needs and capacities define.

- *Individuality:* to be self-differentiating, see and know one's uniqueness, verify the existence and identity of oneself, distinguish self from others, and confirm the entitlement of one's interests, skills, and differences.

- *Affiliation:* to have evidence of belonging; be part of a dyad, group, or cluster; have associations with others; and know interdependence.

- *Volition:* to have alternatives, access to sufficient information, and latitude to make and act on one's choice.

- *Consensual validation:* to have feedback from one's activity and from other people that verifies one's perceptions and reality and to be part of reciprocal exchanges that clarify and acknowledge one's contributions and actions.

- *Predictability:* to discern and evaluate cause and effect and to be able to predict, limit ambiguity, and chanciness, give order to one's world, and experience the comfort of predictable.

- *Self-efficacy:* to have evidence of one's competence, of being able to cope and manage one's everyday life, of being a cause, and of making things happen.

- *Adventure:* to seek and try out the new, the unknown; to explore; to look beyond the here and now; and to discover, experiment, and dare to risk.

- *Accommodation:* to be free from physical and mental harm and to function in an environment that is responsive to individual capabilities while compensating for individual limitations.

- *Reflection:* to have respite from activity, ponder on the meaning of things, and review and contemplate recent and past events.

B. Which activities do you suggest should be increased or added? Which ones should be reduced or eliminated? Why?

C. How would you summarize the human needs equation of this environment?

D. Descriptive summary: Develop an overall evaluation of the strengths and limitations of the environment and its related activities from the perspective of human need responsiveness.

REFERENCES

Barker, R. (1963). On the nature of the environment. *Journal of Social Issues, 19,* 17-38.

Beck, A. C., & Hillmar, E. D. (1986). *Positive management practices.* San Francisco: Jossey-Bass.

Bolman, L. C., & Deal, T. E. (1984). *Modern approaches to understanding and managing organizations.* San Francisco: Jossey-Bass.

Corcoran, M., & Gitlin, L. (1997). The role of the environment in occupational performance. In: C. Christiansen & C. Baum (Eds.). *Enabling performance and well being.* Thorofare, NJ: SLACK Incorporated.

Dunn, W., Brown, C., & McGuigan, A. (1994). The ecology of human performance: A framework for considering the affect of context. *Am J Occup Ther, 48*(7), 595-607.

Fidler, G. (1996). Lifestyle performance: From profile to conceptual model. *Am J Occup Ther, 50*(2), 139-147.

Fidler, G., & Bristow, B. (1992). *Recapturing competence. A systems change for geropsychiatric care.* New York: Springer.

Hall, E. T. (1966). *The hidden dimension.* Garden City, NY: Doubleday.

Hersey, P., & Blanchard, K. (1982). *Management of organizational behavior.* Englewood Cliffs, NJ: Prentice Hall.

Kanter, R. M. (1983). *The change masters.* New York: Simon and Schuster.

Kelly, G. R., & Godbey, G. (1992). *Sociology of leisure.* State College, PA: Venture.

Letts, L., Law, M., Rigby, P., et al (1994). Person-environment assessments in occupational therapy. *Am J Occup Ther, 48*(7), 608-617.

Perkins, E. P., & Shoemaker, A. L. (1990). Indoor play environments: Research and design implications. In G. Fein and M. Riukin, *The young child at play.* Washington, DC: National Association for the Education of Young Children.

Senge, P. (1990). *The fifth discipline.* New York: Doubleday.

Spencer, J. C. (1991). The physical environment and performance. In: C. Christiansen & C. Baum (Eds.). *Occupational therapy: Overcoming human performance deficits.* Thorofare, NJ: SLACK Incorporated.

Spivak, M. (1973). Archetypal places. *Architectural Forum, 140,* 48-48.

ADDITIONAL READING

Csikzentmihalyi, M., & Rochberg-Halton, E. (1981). *The meaning of things.* Cambridge: Cambridge University Press.

Davies, P. (1995). Where does time go? *New Statesman and Society, 8*(353), 29-30.

Peters, T. J. & Waterman, R. H. (1982). *In search of excellence: Lessons from America's best run companies.* New York: Harper & Row.

CHAPTER 13

Summary Overview

Gail S. Fidler

As activities are examined, it becomes increasingly clear that meaning and relevance extend well beyond what is evident. Activities are indeed rich in metaphor and symbol. The synthesis of form and structure, objects and action processes of activities symbolize and represent values, attitudes, beliefs, and feelings. Coupled with the realities of these elements, we can begin to understand how and why activities are such a powerful force in human development.

Adaptation is said to exist when there is a congruence, a match between an individual and the environment. Adaptation and coping require sufficient intact sensory, motor, cognitive, and psychological systems that make it possible for the individual to receive and organize stimuli and appropriately respond to the input. We should now be able to understand how activities enable the development and integration of these systems and elicit adaptive responses. Furthermore, we can begin to appreciate the extent to which activity engagement can provide feedback relative to one's current adaptive capacities. The match of activity characteristics to the person or group is, as we can now appreciate, crucial in this process. The use of task-oriented groups, for example, over a prolonged period of time (Fidler, 1968) has made it possible for me to hypothesize a relationship between the tasks chosen by a group and the level and nature of a group's concerns, progress, and coping skills. For instance, a young adult male group grappling with problems related to parental role expectations, identity, and responsibilities chose to cook, making candies and cakes for themselves. After a period of time, the group discussed the possibility of a cook-out steak dinner with a few selected guests. The ensuing discussions left little doubt that preparing a steak dinner for guests had meaning beyond a steak being a steak. A spaghetti dinner for themselves was the alternative, with the steak cook-out occurring later in the life of the group. From chocolate and sweets, to spaghetti, to steak, to self, then others was a symbolic profile of this group's learning and development.

In another setting, an adult group chose to make a doll house for a local pediatric center. The problems that arose in this process, the "horse play," fantasies, and growing up reminiscences that ensued with the construction of each room, the inordinate attachment to this project, the care and concern for it, the notable reluctance to give it away, seemed clearly related to their own growing up experiences, their here and now needs and concerns. The activity was a symbolic ontogenetic recapitulation.

In still another quite different situation, a 7-year-old boy's behavior was creating concern at a public playground. He was spending most of his time vigorously throwing stones, posing a threat to other children as well as staff. On observation, it appeared that his throwing was not random. Rather, he seemed to be taking careful aim at objects, testing his accuracy. Additionally, his body movement seemed to signal a high level of physical energy and fluid coordinated movement. Providing the boy with a tennis racket and ball, challenging him to hit the ball against the clubhouse wall, brought about what playground staff saw as a "miracle." His stone throwing stopped abruptly, replaced by a persistent, vigorous racquet skill practice. Ultimately, a teenage boy was enlisted to teach him the game of tennis, which he mastered exceptionally well. He was further challenged by us to best his own time in runs around the perimeter of the playground. Testing and competing with himself in addition to discovering and using his physical skills was a remarkable experience for this young boy. As he matured, he became a credible tennis player and long distance runner.

The group of kite flying executives and the story of Mary described by Fidler and Fidler (1983) are further examples of the dynamic interplay of reality and symbol in activities and the critical significance of matching characteristics to person. Csikszentmihalyi (1990) so eloquently describes this process of connectedness with activity, with doing. His scholarly work gives us a magnificent view of the subjectivity of engagement in doing.

Assessing situations, making decisions, and appropriately responding are essential parts of coping and adaptation. The ability to act with purpose is a necessary function of living. Volition, the act of exercising one's will or intention, has been described as a process that involves being aware of alternatives, assessing these, making a choice, planning action on the basis of such choice, inhibiting extraneous stimuli, and acting by following through on one's plan (Arieti, 1967; Kielhofner, 1985). The relationship of these processes to both the real and symbolic characteristics of an activity is certainly evident.

When more than the verbal realm is involved, when touch, hearing, vision, and kinetics are all called into active play, there is, of course, a keener sense of being engaged, of being a cause. Feedback from one's action is immediate, observable, and available for reflection and retrial (Fidler & Fidler, 1978; Pribram, 1971). Verification of being able to make things happen is less obscure, and casual relationships are more obvious.

Activities and occupations involve simultaneously realistic and symbolic experiences of performing, producing, managing, controlling, manipulating, creating, causing to happen, putting in order, and sequencing. These all relate to varying aspects of perception and cognition, assessing and confronting reality, validating one's ideas or intentions, defining the parameters of one's influence, integrating feelings, thoughts, and actions, organizing one's responses, managing time, exercising volition, and verifying one's ability to have some influence on and some control over the events in one's life. Such productive human action, whether it is manifested in a specific project, learning or perfecting a skill, or contributing to a team or group effort, provides a microcosm of life situations. In producing and responding to objects, the individual brings into being his or her individuality and, through choices of response, learns a range of attitudes and behaviors relevant to coping and adaptation (Fidler, 1968).

Menuhin (1969) artfully expresses the essence of activity engagement when he writes,

> *Until we can restore the spontaneous elation that comes of one's efforts with one's own capabilities—respond to a piece of wood—a sheet of paper—a length of cloth or leather or upon one's own mind as does the philosopher, or upon one's own physique as does the dancer; until a substantial proportion of one population is acquainted with the sensations of artistic endeavor we will not satisfactorily overcome the debasement of human values.* (p. 170)

With a deepened knowledge of activities, both our vision and capacities will broaden. Such knowledge will make it possible to create doing environments that will enhance human performance, nurture wellness, and deepen the quality of living. Coming to truly understand and acquiring a sophisticated appreciation for the meaning and relevance of activities, of occupation to the evolution of a positive regard for self and others, to adaptation, to living, and to the quality of that living may make it possible for us to begin to develop a science, fashion an art of practice, and shape an identity worthy of the concept of doing as the enabler of human performance and as the essence of the quality of life.

References

Arieti, S. (1967). *The intrapsychic self*. New York: Basic Books.

Csikszentmihalyi, M. (1990). *Flow: The psychology of optimal experience*. New York: Harper Row.

Fidler, G. S. (1968). The task oriented group as a context for treatment. *Am J Occup Ther, 23*, 43-48.

Fidler, G. S. (1981). From crafts to competence. *Am J Occup Ther, 35*, 567-573.

Fidler, G. S. & Fidler J. W. (1978). Doing and becoming: Purposeful action and self-actualization. *Am J Occup Ther, 32*, 305-310.

Fidler, G. S. & Fidler, J. W. (1983). Doing and becoming: The occupational therapy experience. In: G. Kielhofner (Ed.). *Health through occupation: Theory and practice in occupational therapy,* pp. 267-280. Philadelphia: F. A. Davis

Kielhofner, G. (1985). *A model of human occupation: Theory and application*. Baltimore: Williams & Wilkins.

Menuhin, Y. (1969). Music and the nature of its contribution to humanity. In: D. Hayman. *The arts and man*. New York: Prentice Hall.

Pribram, K. H. (1971). *Language of the brain*. Englewood Cliffs, NJ: Prentice Hall.

Additional Reading

Kielhofner, G. (1997). *Conceptual foundations of occupational therapy*. Philadelphia: F. A. Davis.

INDEX

BUILD *Your Library*

This book and many others on numerous different topics are available from SLACK Incorporated. For further information or a copy of our latest catalog, contact us at:

Professional Book Division
SLACK Incorporated
6900 Grove Road
Thorofare, NJ 08086 USA
Telephone: 1-856-848-1000
1-800-257-8290
Fax: 1-856-853-5991
E-mail: orders@slackinc.com
www.slackinc.com

We accept most major credit cards and checks or money orders in US dollars drawn on a US bank. Most orders are shipped within 72 hours.

Contact us for information on recent releases, forthcoming titles, and bestsellers. If you have a comment about this title or see a need for a new book, direct your correspondence to the Editorial Director at the above address.

Thank you for your interest and we hope you found this work beneficial.